Information and Communication Technologies in Behavioral Health

A Literature Review with Recommendations for the Air Force

Joshua Breslau, Charles C. Engel

RAND Project AIR FORCE

Prepared for the United States Air Force
Approved for public release; distribution unlimited

RAND CORPORATION

For more information on this publication, visit www.rand.org/t/RR1054

Library of Congress Cataloging-in-Publication Data is available for this publication.

ISBN: 978-0-8330-9012-6

Published by the RAND Corporation, Santa Monica, Calif.

Preface

Over the past decade, dramatic growth in information and communication technologies (ICTs), many now active on users' smartphones 24 hours a day, has led to rapid innovation in methods for providing behavioral health care. A recent RAND study found that these innovations are already having a wide impact within the U.S. Air Force, with nearly half of airmen reporting use of ICTs to access behavioral health information. Developing a strategy for navigating this new arena of health technology that acknowledges its promises and pitfalls is particularly important for the Air Force, given the focus on behavioral health consequences of the conflicts in Iraq and Afghanistan. To inform strategy related to ICTs for behavioral health, the Air Force Surgeon General asked RAND Project AIR FORCE (PAF) to review the scientific literature on their use and efficacy.

For the purposes of developing this strategy, we review the literature following a public health model that distinguishes between two major types of ICTs being used to improve behavioral health:

1. ICTs are being introduced in nonclinical, preventive interventions that aim to address large populations. These uses can be universal, addressing individuals regardless of their characteristics, or they can be targeted, designed specifically for an identifiable high-risk group.
2. ICTs are also being introduced into clinical treatment for individuals who have initiated treatment with a provider. Some ICTs have been developed as supplements to clinical treatment, and others have been developed to take the place of in-person treatment as the primary modality of treatment.

In this report, we review the evidence for the potential uses of ICTs across the spectrum of public health interventions, describing the available technologies and reviewing the scientific literature for evidence of efficacy.

The research reported here was sponsored by the Air Force Surgeon General and conducted within the Manpower, Personnel, and Training Program of PAF.

RAND Project AIR FORCE

RAND Project AIR FORCE, a division of the RAND Corporation, is the U.S. Air Force's federally funded research and development center for studies and analyses. PAF provides the Air Force with independent analyses of policy alternatives affecting the development, employment, combat readiness, and support of current and future air, space, and cyber forces. Research is conducted in four programs: Force Modernization and Employment; Manpower, Personnel, and

Training; Resource Management; and Strategy and Doctrine. The research reported here was prepared under contract FA7014-06-C-0001.

Additional information about PAF is available on our website:
http://www.rand.org/paf/

Table of Contents

Figures and Tables

Figures

Tables

Summary

The growth in information and communication technologies (ICTs) has led to rapid innovation in methods for providing behavioral health care, a wide field of services including prevention and treatment of both substance use and psychiatric disorders. Innovations range from updating and enhancing older technologies, such as electronic health records and telemedicine, to the thousands of mental health–related applications now available on smartphones. These innovations have created new opportunities to improve the quality of mental health care, expand access to mental health information, enable new methods for providing care, encourage patient adherence to treatment, and even reduce the stigma often associated with seeking treatment.

The challenge, however, lies in determining what functions ICTs should fill in mental health service delivery and gaining insight into the effectiveness of the many available tools. While thousands of apps are available, there is little guidance available to users or mental health professionals about which tools and programs are the most promising. A growing gap exists between the availability of ICTs and scientific evidence to inform the use of these tools in mental health service delivery. Addressing this gap is particularly important to the U.S. military in light of recent involvement in the prolonged armed conflicts in Iraq and Afghanistan and the subsequent focus on behavioral health consequences for U.S. military personnel.

ICTs may represent a strategic opportunity to improve access to mental health information and assistance. Motivated by a desire to better understand this landscape and, particularly, the research supporting the use of ICTs for providing mental health care, the U.S. Air Force Surgeon General asked RAND Project AIR FORCE to conduct a literature review about the use of ICTs to help answer the following questions:

- When is their use most effective?
- Do they improve the quality and effectiveness of care?
- Can they improve patient adherence to treatment?
- What are the costs and benefits?
- What considerations must be given to incorporating these methods into military care options?

This report provides the results of that review.

RAND used a commonly referenced public health model of the clinical process for providing mental health care as an organizing construct for the use of ICTs (Figure S.1). The foundation of the model is universal prevention interventions that address the entire population. Next are targeted prevention interventions that aim to reach people who are known to have a high risk of or predisposition toward mental health problems that could lead to adverse outcomes. Clinical interventions, represented by the top of the triangle, include all the treatment provided in the formal health care system to individuals with clinical conditions. RAND addressed the use of ICTs in each of these settings.

Figure S.1. Public Health Model for ICT Uses in Behavioral Health

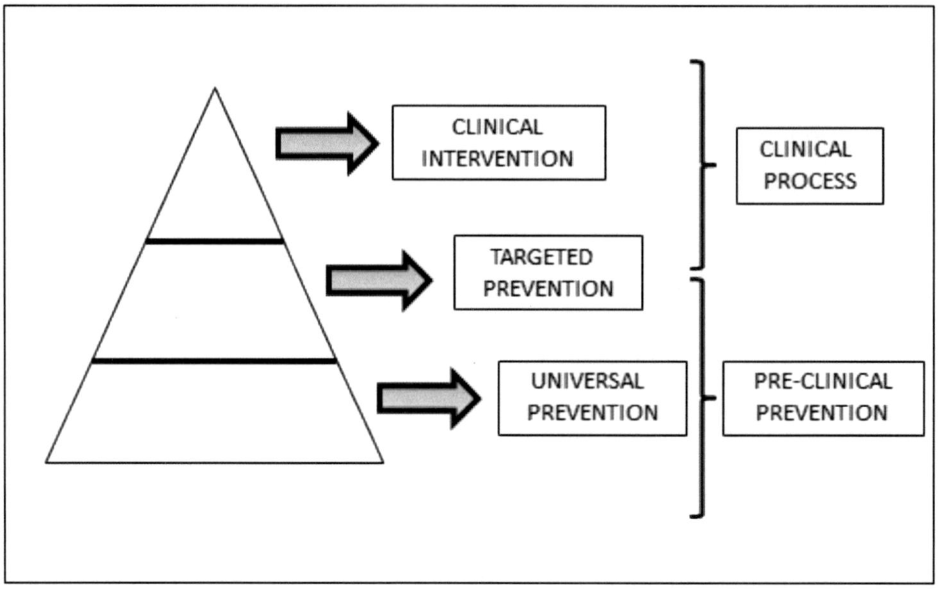

SOURCE: Adapted from Frieden, 2010.

Prevention

Prevention is a preclinical or clinical activity that involves averting some aspect of an illness before it occurs. The literature suggests potential strategies for applying ICTs to universal prevention (efforts that address the entire population without respect to individuals' preexisting level of risk, including personalized assessment of behavioral health risk factors) and targeted prevention (efforts focused on a specific at-risk group, including delivery of information tailored to individuals with particular health risks). Preventive ICTs use such new technological forms as online education, supportive therapies, the use of email or text-based communication while deployed, and smartphone or video-linked social support tools. Potential applications include depression, anxiety, posttraumatic stress symptoms (PTSS), substance misuse, and intimate partner problems.

Although the level of evidence from published and scientifically valid research trials supporting the preventive use of ICTs for these problems is scarce, some low-cost, low-risk opportunities exist. Education efforts are generally seen as a public good, and the demand for efficacy and safety data is low. Efforts to use the Internet, smartphone apps, and similar technologies to increase Air Force and family member understanding of mental health issues and reduce the mystery and stigma that surround them are responsible and well advised, but these efforts should be considered in light of the resources needed to sustain them. There is currently little scientific evidence supporting additional investment in ICT-based psychosocial programs for resilience or prevention of PTSS, depression, or anxiety. Instead, preventive interventions might prioritize problems of alcohol misuse and intimate partner violence (IPV). Given the unique features and needs of the Air Force population, any effort to implement preventive behavioral health ICTs will necessitate ongoing monitoring of program safety and effectiveness.

Clinical Treatment

The clinical process begins with the initial contact between a patient and a care provider. ICT interventions associated with the clinical process may be used for patient education and activation, to improve decisionmaking by clinicians, to provide a therapy, to improve adherence to treatment, or to maintain treatment gains over time. ICT applications that can be used to support the clinical process occupy a rapidly changing area of technology development, and research on the efficacy of specific ICT applications cannot keep up with their evolution. The literature is vast, but much of it is descriptive or based on uncontrolled observational studies, making it difficult to draw conclusions regarding how these tools might best be used.

Despite the lack of solid research evidence to date, ICTs hold promise in addressing the challenges of mental health care. ICTs offer an advance in convenience for providers and clinicians, which can be advantageous in the military, with its frequent moves and inflexible schedules. One promising avenue is development of reliable methods for patient-clinician communication between therapy sessions; another is Internet-based cognitive behavioral therapy. Even if off-the-shelf products are not available, the success described in the literature suggests that these should be priority target areas for Air Force efforts. How ICT applications developed for particular target populations might translate into a military environment is an area that will need further investigation and should be one component in developing an ICT implementation strategy. Cost trade-offs are another area that needs further study within the military community to determine what level of use justifies the investment.

Recommendations

ICTs offer a wide range of innovative techniques designed to improve access to behavioral health care and to improve the quality of care that is delivered. The evidence to date on effectiveness and efficiency of use is vast but uneven, and how these research results apply to the population of airmen in the U.S. Air Force is unclear. Much of the research focuses on the use of ICTs to extend services to individuals already in clinical treatment. Yet this research offers little insight into how those tools might scale up for use in preventive care that is targeted toward a far larger population. For this larger population, the available research is much more limited and fails to address such important concerns as safety, adverse effects, and inconsistent results. Furthermore, there is little or no evidence in the literature regarding the efficacy of some of the most recently developed types of ICTs, in particular those using smartphones.

Despite its limitations, the literature does offer constructive lessons and opportunities that can inform the development of a responsible strategy for implementing behavioral health ICTs. Our recommendations focus on ICT strategies for the Air Force rather than specific applications that can be immediately put into place. In our judgment, the Air Force should take an incremental approach to adopting the use of these tools—one that involves a program of measurement-based implementation and process and outcome monitoring rather than urgent dissemination. The most significant concerns surrounding a more aggressive approach to implementation are efficient use of resources and the safety, privacy, and applicability of existing behavioral health ICTs in the Air Force.

General Recommendations

We offer a number of general recommendations toward developing an effective Air Force strategy:

1. **The Air Force should develop and adopt a coordinated interdisciplinary strategy for behavioral health ICT implementation.** Just as important as the question of which ICTs should be used and how and where to use them is the strategy employed for managing emerging health technologies. In developing this strategy, the Air Force should work with an interdisciplinary mix of professionals with behavioral health, public health, information technology, mental health measurement, and health communications expertise.
2. **The Air Force should develop standards and objectives for adapting ICTs to the unique Air Force context and implement a method for determining when the standard has been met before fielding a given ICT.** Most available tools have been tested in a nonmilitary setting. Field testing in a military environment will be needed to reduce unintended organizational and health consequences and maximize benefits for the intended populations and individuals.
3. **Air Force behavioral health ICTs should be designed for monitoring aggregate use and intervention outcomes, including adverse or unintended effects.** An advantage of ICTs, apart from their potential to improve health and prevent health problems, is the potential for transparent, built-in measurement features. Behavioral health ICTs are medical devices. In a manner consistent with continuous quality improvement programs in the clinical service delivery domain, establishing the ongoing safety and effectiveness of these ICT-based programs of care is necessary for ongoing, responsible use.

The report also details a number of specific recommendations regarding the use of ICTs in the prevention and treatment of behavioral health problems.

Prevention Recommendations

1. **If the Air Force introduces ICTs for prevention, it should review existing ICTs provided to airmen across the Department of Defense (DoD), the services, and supporting private organizations to harmonize efforts with existing programs.** There are ongoing efforts in a variety of military, governmental, and private sources. The

potential for duplication of efforts is great without careful ongoing review, particularly because there is no comprehensive, up-to-date list of preventive behavioral health programs or ICTs.

2. **The Air Force should seek and collate aggregate search engine data from Air Force and DoD websites aiming to provide preventive assistance to airmen and families.** Search terms may be a simple, low-cost way of identifying the interests and needs of the Air Force population and enhancing web-based information resources for airmen and their families.
3. **The Air Force should not use ICTs for the purpose of targeting traumatized units or individuals for "critical incident stress debriefings" or "psychological debriefings."** Extensive research relating to interventions to prevent PTSS and posttraumatic stress disorder (PTSD) is clear. These interventions, particularly when mandated, do not prevent PTSS symptoms, and there is no evidence to suggest that currently available technologies offer a new way forward in this preventive area.
4. **The Air Force should consider adapting and implementing ICTs offering Internet-based, personalized single-session feedback for airmen at identified risk for future alcohol-related incidents.** Alcohol misuse is a common problem in the military and a major factor in IPV and preventable and fatal injuries, including suicide. The Internet offers low-cost opportunities to deliver this preventive intervention in ways that are accountable and assess for general effectiveness.
5. **The Air Force should consider the use of ICTs for universal and targeted prevention efforts relating to IPV.** About half of airmen are married, and a much larger proportion are involved in intimate partner relationships. At least one universal preventive ICT approach, ePREP, is well studied and effective for preventing IPV.

Clinical Treatment Recommendations

1. **The Air Force should adopt an Internet-based treatment program for depression and anxiety, tailored to the needs of the Air Force population.** An Internet-based cognitive behavioral therapy program could fill a niche in the mental health care delivery system by providing a treatment option for airmen who are remote from treatment, highly mobile, or concerned about the stigma of attending a mental health clinic. Procedures for guaranteeing confidentiality of treatment, particularly if treatment enables patient-physician contact via smartphone, should be in place prior to the introduction of new Internet-based treatment programs.
2. **The Air Force should monitor the future development of Internet-based treatments for substance misuse.** Although no off-the-shelf programs in this area offer proven efficacy, there are a number of promising recently developed programs, such as brief interventions for alcohol misuse, that could prove valuable to the Air Force.
3. **The Air Force should select smartphone apps that airmen can use to monitor their medication use and communicate with mental health clinicians between in-person visits.** For both of these functions, evidence suggests that smartphone apps provide effective tools that make adherence to treatment more convenient. Given the large number of apps currently available, the selection of specific apps will require an

extensive review of existing options and particular attention to the ability of clinicians to ensure the confidentiality of treatment-related information for their patients.

The rapidly changing field of ICT applications for mental health care promises to improve treatment systems in ways that address long-standing problems in both the civilian and military service systems. However, very few ICT applications have moved from promising to proven technologies. Only a small handful of ICT applications, notably those designed for Internet cognitive behavioral therapy, are supported by evidence-based research. Nonetheless, other ICTs appear to be promising based on the convenience and efficiency they add to established evidence-based treatments and evidence of their acceptability to patients and providers. Over time, the research literature and clinical experience with ICTs will grow, and consensus will form on which ICT applications are of greatest benefit to patients.

Acknowledgments

We thank the Air Force action officers and advisors in the Air Force Surgeon General's office who provided earlier feedback on the literature review: Col Tracy Neal-Walden, Col Kathleen Crimmons, Maj Nicole Fuller, and Velda Johnson. This manuscript benefited from the editorial assistance of Barbara Bicksler. Ray Conley, Kirsten Keller, and Laura Miller offered suggestions for improvement on an earlier draft of this manuscript.

Abbreviations

CBT	cognitive behavioral therapy
CCDS	computerized clinical decision support
CSF	[Army] Comprehensive Soldier Fitness
DoD	U.S. Department of Defense
HIE	health information exchange
iCBT	Internet cognitive behavioral therapy
ICT	information and communication technology
IMCP	interactive multimedia computer program
IoM	Institute of Medicine
IPV	intimate partner violence
PTSD	posttraumatic stress disorder
PTSS	posttraumatic stress symptoms
RCT	randomized controlled trial
SHUTi	Sleep Healthy Using the Internet
VA	U.S. Department of Veterans Affairs

1. Background

Over the past decade, the development and diffusion of information and communication technologies (ICTs) have led to rapid innovation in methods for providing behavioral health care, a broad category of care that includes prevention and treatment of both substance use and psychiatric disorders. These innovations include extensions of older technologies, such as electronic health records and telemedicine, as well as wholly new methods for providing care through channels only recently made available by the pervasive use of smartphones. In January 2014, a search for mental health–related apps found 5,181 apps available on the Google Play site and 1,766 apps available on the Apple App Store (Table 1.1). While this rapid innovation in technology has the potential to improve access to mental health information and enable new methods for providing care, there is still a great deal of uncertainty about the specific functions that ICTs can and should fill in mental health service delivery. Moreover, there is wide variation in the quality of ICT apps in mental health and little guidance available to individual users, mental health professionals, or health policy decisionmakers that can help identify the most promising new programs.

Table 1.1. Number of Behavioral-Health-Related Apps on the Google and Apple App Stores, January 2014

Search Term	Google Play	Apple App Store
Depression	1,615	586
Anxiety	1,269	775
Schizophrenia	67	20
Bipolar	151	90
Psychiatry	168	149
Alcoholism	1,911	146

SOURCE: Chan et al., 2014.

There is no question that the rapid expansion of ICTs has created new opportunities for mental health care. According to the Pew Research Internet Project (2014), 58 percent of American adults owned a smartphone (i.e., an Internet-connected mobile phone) in January 2014, with much higher proportions in younger age groups: 74 percent in the 30–49 age group and 83 percent in the 18–29 age group. Among airmen, most of whom fall into the younger age groups, the patterns are similar. A recent Project AIR FORCE study (Miller et al., 2014) found that most airmen report using some form of ICT every day for either work or nonwork purposes.

For work purposes, nearly 80 percent of airmen reported using email daily, over 60 percent reported daily phone use, 28 percent used Internet daily for work purposes, and over 10 percent texted messages every day. For nonwork purposes, 70 percent of airmen reported daily texting, 60 percent reported daily phone use, and 45 percent used social networking or other Internet sites daily. Forty-three percent of airmen have used ICTs to find mental health–related information.

This report addresses the gap between the rapid growth in availability of ICTs for mental health and the lack of information regarding the evidence base for using these new technologies in mental health service delivery. Addressing this gap is particularly important in light of U.S. military involvement in the prolonged armed conflicts in Iraq and Afghanistan and the focus of news media and research attention on behavioral health consequences for U.S. military personnel. ICTs may represent a strategic opportunity to improve access to mental health information and assistance. Recognizing the potential opportunity, the U.S. Air Force Surgeon General asked RAND Project AIR FORCE to conduct a literature review guided by the following questions:

1. Can mental health care providers use ICTs to improve the quality and effectiveness of the care they provide to their patients?
2. Are there some types of problems better or equally addressed through ICTs and some that should only be done face to face?
3. How can ICTs improve patient adherence to mental health treatment?
4. Have care options through ICTs enabled mental health professionals to provide care for individuals who otherwise would not have been willing to obtain face-to-face counseling? If so, what do we know about those individuals' demographic characteristics, diagnoses, and hurdles to receiving face-to-face care?

To address these issues, RAND researchers undertook a review of the scientific literature evaluating the application of ICTs to mental health care delivery. We present the results of this review following a public health intervention model described below. Based on the literature review, in the final chapter we present recommendations for how the Air Force could incorporate ICTs into the existing mental health care delivery system.

Priority Behavioral Health Issues

This report focuses on a limited number of specific behavioral health issues that were identified as high-priority issues by the Air Force. The priority issues were selected not only because of their immediate health burden but also because of their connection to multiple adverse outcomes among airmen. Specifically, we focus on the following issues:

1. depressive symptoms, including but not limited to major depression
2. substance misuse, particularly alcohol misuse

3. intimate partner relationship issues
4. posttraumatic stress symptoms (PTSS), including but not limited to posttraumatic stress disorder (PTSD).

These priority issues were selected not only because of their immediate health burden but also because of their connection to multiple adverse outcomes among airmen. For instance, alcohol misuse is a contributing factor in a wide range of incidents, including motor vehicle accidents and interpersonal violence. Improving treatment of these priority issues is considered strategic for their potential benefits across this range of adverse outcomes.

The Promise of ICTs in Mental Health Care

A wide range of potential uses for ICTs in mental health care have been envisioned by researchers and technology developers (A. M. Bauer et al., 2014; Donker et al., 2013; Luxton et al., 2011; Mohr et al., 2013a). Some ICT applications in mental health use Internet-connected computers, while many of the most recently developed applications take advantage of the ubiquity of smartphones and their ability to systematically collect, analyze, and transmit data. Technology in every smartphone can be used to monitor an individual's location and movement, assess his or her mental health status over time, provide timely mental health information, and communicate with clinicians. These functions offer the promise of addressing at least four major limitations of the existing mental health system:

1. **Quality of care.** Research in civilian health systems has found that quality of care for mental health problems rarely meets the standards set by agreed-upon clinical guidelines (Price et al., 2013; Varshney, 2014). ICT applications built into electronic health record systems can address this issue by analyzing patient medical history, prompting clinicians to screen for mental health problems, aiding the clinician in differential diagnosis and treatment planning, and tracking patient progress over time.
2. **Access to care.** In rural or remote areas, access to mental health care is frequently limited. Often this means that the only option for patients is to seek care from nonspecialist clinicians—e.g., in primary care clinics—rather than from mental health specialists who are better prepared to provide evidence-based clinical treatments. ICTs offer the potential for clinicians to provide treatment remotely, either face to face using telemedicine or through the Internet using Internet-based treatments (Clarke and Yarborough, 2013; Bennett and Glasgow, 2009).
3. **Treatment dropout.** Once patients make contact with a clinician and begin a course of treatment for a mental health problem, dropout prior to completion of a standard course of treatment is extremely common. ICTs promise methods for patients and therapists to continue communication between in-person visits so that patients remain engaged in treatment and are less likely to drop out (Krishna, Boren, and Balas, 2009; Fiordelli, Diviani, and Schulz, 2013).

4. **Treatment stigma.** The stigma of mental illness, which can be particularly acute in military settings, is a significant barrier to mental health treatment. The ability to access care through an ICT in private, rather than in a clinic that requires some degree of public exposure, may bring more patients in need of care into treatment (Klasnja and Pratt, 2012).

What Are the Challenges?

As with any promising new technology, the utility of ICTs should be evaluated with respect to their ability to improve the delivery of care relative to the existing care system. This requires balancing the promised advantages of an ICT application against a number of potentially countervailing effects. Specific issues related to particular ICTs will be discussed in detail in the body of the report, but four general issues are important to consider because they are likely to apply to many proposed ICT applications:

1. **Uptake.** A critical issue with respect to most ICTs, particularly those involved in direct clinical care, is whether the population for which they are intended will actually use them. Uptake is often difficult to estimate even for well-studied applications because efficacy studies are often not designed to be informative about uptake in real-world situations. For instance, a randomized trial that compared in-person treatment to ICT-based treatment typically will only include individuals who are motivated to begin the treatment in question. While the ICT-based treatment may be comparable in efficacy to the in-person treatment, the trial will not provide evidence that implementation of the ICT-based treatment will expand the population receiving treatment beyond those who are already motivated to start it. This distinction between efficacy and uptake is important to consider, given the goal of using ICTs to expand the population reach of effective mental health treatment.
2. **Quality of care.** Although ICTs promise improvements in quality of care, there has also been a persistent concern with their ability to maintain quality, with respect to both the information and care that they provide. As noted above, thousands of apps purport to provide mental health information or to support mental health treatment. Yet in many cases, it is difficult to evaluate the quality of the information being provided or the effectiveness with which the information is presented. While some apps are created or endorsed by trusted professional organizations, many are of uncertain origin with questionable credibility. Many apps are created by private for-profit businesses that may have little interest in pursuing evidenced-based evaluations of their content or efficacy. Regardless of the credibility of the source, apps may not present information in a way that aligns with the level of electronic health literacy in the target population (A. M. Bauer et al., 2014). The variable quality of ICTs makes it important for leadership to help airmen identify the most helpful and trustworthy resources, given that they are already using ICTs in large numbers. Moreover, where ICTs extend access to services, such as crisis intervention, quality of care will depend more on the existing system of care than on the ICT itself.
3. **Privacy.** ICTs may introduce threats to the privacy of protected health information that are less pronounced in traditional in-person treatment. For instance, when protected

health information is transmitted between patients and clinicians, the transmission must comply with federal laws (e.g., the Health Insurance Portability and Accountability Act of 1996) (Lawley, 2012). ICTs can also raise new issues, such as determining the identity of the patient or the clinician during an encounter. Using a smartphone, a user's identity cannot be confirmed if the communication is by text. However, much more certainty is provided by videoconferencing applications in which the clinician and patient can see each other. Smartphones may store sensitive information in ways that users do not know how to access or protect, such as records of texts sent or received, and users may use their smartphone apps in settings in which their confidentiality is compromised without their awareness, such as a dorm room, barracks, or coffee shop. Data mining for commercial purposes may put patients who receive care through the Internet at additional risk.

4. **Costs.** While the costs of ICTs are generally thought to be considerably less than those associated with traditional in-person mental health services, there are important aspects to consider. Costs may include training staff to support ICT-based services, adapting software to meet the specific needs of a program, purchases of computer hardware and software, and licensing fees. For instance, an Internet-based treatment program may be simple to offer, but the low uptake may not justify shifting resources from existing in-person services.

Theoretical Model of the Clinical Process in Behavioral Health

A public health model of the clinical process for providing mental health care guided this review. In selecting this model, our goal was to give priority to the delivery system function an ICT might enhance. This approach, starting with the need rather than the technology, helps to focus attention on ways that ICTs can enhance the efficiency of existing health services. As shown in Figure 1.1, the public health model views health interventions along a continuum from universal prevention to targeted prevention to clinical intervention. Universal prevention interventions, at the base of the triangle, address the entire population, without regard to each individual's level of risk. These interventions may aim to educate as many people as possible about an issue in order to affect social norms in the culture, and they are generally the least costly per individual reached. Targeted prevention interventions are similar in that they aim to reach people who have not yet been identified as having a specific medical need, but they address a specific portion of the population, usually one known to be at high risk. Clinical interventions, represented by the top of the triangle, include all the treatment provided in the formal health care system to individuals with identified clinical conditions. Clinical interventions are the most expensive to provide, and they reach the smallest and most ill segment of the population.

Figure 1.1. Public Health Model for ICT Uses in Behavioral Health

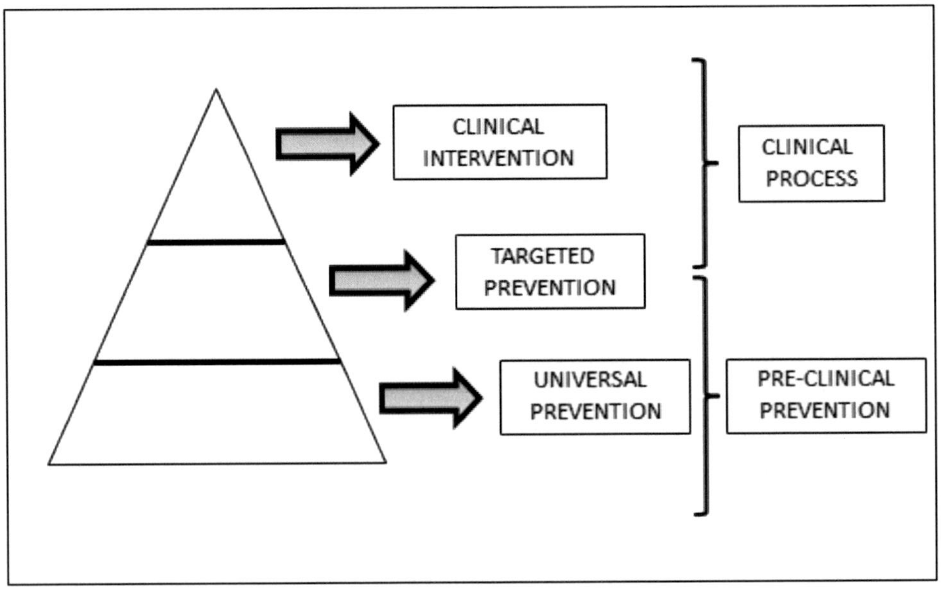

SOURCE: Adapted from Frieden, 2010.

This public health model can be broken down into preclinical and clinical components and further into subcomponents. The preclinical components are those that precede identification of a specific mental health problem and include universal preventive measures, such as educational programming and targeted dissemination of support tools. All of these preclinical components are preventive in nature. The clinical process begins with the initial contact between a patient and a care provider and can involve prevention or treatment of mental or behavioral health problems. Interventions addressing this component, shown in Figure 1.2, may be provided in the waiting room prior to an actual clinical encounter, they may be provided during a clinical encounter as a treatment support to the clinician or the patient, or they may replace a clinical encounter, moving the primary treatment process into an ICT channel. Finally, ICTs may also be used to maintain therapeutic gains after completion of a course of treatment, a particularly important function for psychiatric disorders that tend to be chronic and intermittent in nature.

Figure 1.2. Clinical Public Health Interventions

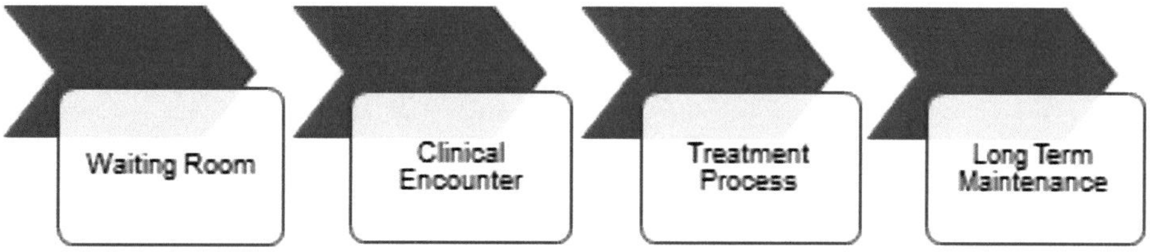

Evaluating the Evidence

Given the broad scope of this review and the many possible interventions using ICTs in mental health care, it is important to consider how the research evidence should evaluated. Three particular issues should be considered. First, mental health treatment systems are complex, and the ICTs developed to improve them are highly specialized to those settings (Cheung and Duan, 2014). Evidence based on testing an ICT in one setting may not generalize to a different population or health system. Generalizability is particularly important to consider in drawing lessons for the Air Force based on the civilian literature.

Second, the quality and quantity of research on the full range of ICT applications for mental health treatment is highly variable. For some applications, there are literally hundreds of studies that have already been extensively reviewed and synthesized in the literature. However, for some of the most recently developed types of ICTs, in particular those using smartphones, there is little or no evidence in the literature regarding efficacy. Since studies of these ICTs have not been conducted, beyond feasibility and acceptability studies in a small number of cases, empirical evidence for or against their use is simply not available.

Third, the pace of innovation in ICT applications for behavioral health is much faster than the pace of research that can evaluate the efficacy of those applications (Mohr et al., 2013b). While evidence from multiple randomized controlled trials (RCTs) is required for robust evidence of efficacy, the conduct of a single RCT takes multiple years. ICTs change so rapidly that by the time evidence accumulates for the efficacy of a specific ICT application, that ICT application may have become obsolete. For this reason, measuring the usage of ICTs by clinicians and patients is particularly important, as these measures may provide the only data that can be used to evaluate and update ICT strategies.

In light of these limitations of the literature, this report focuses on identifying ICT *strategies* for the Air Force rather than specific applications that can immediately be put into practice. To that end, the literature review methodology followed a model of the potential clinical applications of ICTs to mental health treatment, aiming to identify those applications where evidence is currently strongest. Narrative reviews of evidence were conducted in each domain identified by the model focusing both on potential applications of ICTs that have been described in theoretical papers and on existing ICTs for which there is empirical research literature. A consensus regarding the current state of knowledge in each domain was reached through discussion between the authors of this report. Consideration was also given to the relevant clinical literature on traditional, in-person treatments within each domain. The report summarized our consensus regarding the implications of the current evidence base for applications of ICTs to mental health treatment in the Air Force. In each area where we make recommendations, we specify the types of evidence that are currently available to support that recommendation, but we also emphasize that in most cases additional work on tailoring ICTs to the Air Force context will be required to achieve the desired benefits.

Organization of the Report

This report discusses the potential applications of ICTs to behavioral care as they have been described and studied in the scientific literature, following the public health model. The second chapter reviews applications of ICTs to universal and targeted prevention of mental health problems, while the third chapter reviews applications of ICTs to clinical treatment. Although the divide between prevention and treatment is not always completely clear, for the purposes of this report we consider any ICT designed to help someone who has already made contact with a clinician as a clinical application instead of a preventive application. In the fourth and final chapter, we draw out recommendations based on the existing literature for an Air Force strategy to make the best use of existing ICTs in mental health treatment and remain apprised of continuing developments in the future.

2. Prevention: Universal and Targeted Approaches

Prevention is a preclinical or clinical activity that involves averting some aspect of an illness before it occurs. For the purpose of this review, we have divided preventive efforts into those that are universal in population scope (which we refer to as *universal prevention*) and those that are targeted to subpopulations with specific risk factors or identified preventive needs (which we refer to as *targeted prevention*). Preventive interventions, particularly those that target specific risk factors, may be clinical or nonclinical in nature. Here, we focus on aspects of prevention that are largely nonclinical, though ICTs may offer unique opportunities to link pre- and nonclinical activities to clinical care in automated ways that, until recently, were technically difficult to achieve. We examine (1) the evidence to support the suggestion that new technologic capabilities of ICTs can produce measurable benefit for populations and individuals and (2) available examples of promising ICTs for use and future testing.

Universal Prevention

Universal prevention is most often aimed at reducing the incidence of a problem—for example, the new onset of a disorder or condition. Ways that an ICT might support universal prevention among military health system beneficiaries include personalized assessment of behavioral health risk factors or delivery of preventive action for individuals determined to be at elevated health risk by a standard assessment. Preventive ICTs may make use of a variety of new technological forms, such as online education, supportive therapies, the use of email- or text-based communication while deployed, or smartphone or video-linked social support tools.

ICTs offer promising opportunities, involve innovative formats, and open up new populations in which service member or family isolation, distress, and psychosocial risk can be decreased. Emerging technologies may

1. help airmen and family members learn about various psychosocial risk factors (e.g., family or personal history of depression, anxiety, or substance misuse; subclinical distress; history of hazardous alcohol use; history of abuse; victim or perpetrator of interpersonal abuse or workplace harassment; chronic health problems, including wounds and injuries)
2. assist in screening for psychosocial risk factors among service members, families, and tracking of symptoms over time
3. bolster social support through the creation of "virtual communities" of support (Welbourne, Blanchard, and Wadsworth, 2013).

Universal Preventive Strategies and the Safety Imperative

Preventive psychosocial approaches are usually viewed as harmless in the worst case and beneficial in most cases. However, it is essential to characterize the potential for harm when seeking to prevent illness in healthy populations. It is important to emphasize that even a program that appears to be "harmless" has opportunity costs; resources devoted to the program are unavailable for other uses that might have beneficial effects.

Unlike targeted preventive or treatment interventions, entire populations are exposed to universal preventive interventions, so it is essential to establish the safety of these interventions. Examples of universal preventive interventions from everyday experience are fluoride in water or seat belt requirements when driving. If a preventive intervention might prevent illness in roughly 10 percent of the population, then it follows that 90 percent of the population cannot benefit from the intervention. These individuals, though we may have no easy way of determining who they are, will remain healthy without prevention. If a preventive treatment could lead to adverse effects, then the risk of exposing an entire population to the treatment can easily outweigh the benefits ultimately received by only 10 percent of the population. This is particularly true if—as is typical for behavioral interventions—the average benefit among the 10 percent is only modest.

Considering adverse effects of preventive psychosocial interventions is critical for a balanced evaluation, and there is increasing awareness that psychosocial interventions in general are not without risk (Rona, Hyams, and Wesseley, 2005). Unfortunately, the safety of these interventions has often been assumed, and therefore few studies of psychological interventions have assessed for or reported adverse events. Jonsson et al. (2014) recently reviewed 132 eligible randomized trials of psychosocial intervention and found that only 28 trials (21 percent) included information indicating that patients had been monitored for adverse effects.

A further challenge to obtaining sound evidence of effectiveness in universal preventive psychosocial trials is the large sample size and long follow-up that these trials require (Muñoz et al., 2010). This too is because most members of the study-eligible population will remain healthy even if the intervention is ineffective. Ironically, however, it is precisely the potential for ICTs to offer preventive assistance to large numbers of people at apparent low cost that makes them an attractive universal preventive possibility.

Universal Prevention Applications for Specific Problems

What then is the state of evidence addressing the use of ICTs in universal population preventive strategies for depression, anxiety, PTSS, substance misuse, and intimate partner problems? In short, a wide range of approaches has been studied, and while the promise these strategies represent is great, thus far the evidence for their effectiveness remains thin.

Depression

Depression is now widely recognized as being among the top five causes of disability both in the United States and globally (McKenna et al., 2005; Whiteford et al., 2013). Muñoz and colleagues (2010) reviewed published randomized trials testing any intervention designed to prevent depression. Of the 29 trials reviewed, only two were universal preventive approaches, and neither involved ICTs. They concluded, based on these studies, that prevention of depression is possible and necessary. However, they emphasized the need to target preventive interventions to groups at relatively high short-term depression risk to ensure that preventive efforts remained feasible and resource efficient. This strategy represents targeted rather than universal prevention and is therefore addressed in subsequent sections of this review.

Posttraumatic Stress Symptoms

The Institute of Medicine (2014) has published a comprehensive review of U.S. Department of Defense (DoD) programs designed to prevent psychological disorders in DoD. The Army's Comprehensive Soldier Fitness (CSF) program is a widely publicized military effort to promote psychosocial resilience and prevent PTSS that involves ICT-based components. The program, designed around Seligman's Penn Resiliency Program (Cornum, Matthews, and Seligman, 2011), aims to prevent psychosocial distress and related loss of function using a positive psychology theoretical framework and intervention applied prior to deployment. Two of the four major CSF components are delivered over the Internet. First, comprehensive resilience components occur through customizable online training modules, addressing topics such as positive psychology; mindfulness; cognitive restructuring; and education on PTSS, occupational health, leadership, deployment, unit cohesion, and the return home after deployment.

Second, the CSF program's ICT-based confidential online assessment tool enabled annual status assessments from program participants. The program has been adapted across the three U.S. military services to include the Air Force's Comprehensive Airman Fitness program (Air Combat Command, undated). In 2009, the Army made an initial $125 million investment in what the Institute of Medicine (IoM) described as "the largest universal prevention program of its kind" (IoM, 2014, p. 128). Indeed, by 2011, it was said to have provided training to over 1 million Army service members.

Lester and colleagues (2011) published pre- and post-assessments of CSF based on a 105-item survey. In that study, the maximum standardized effect size among the outcomes assessed was 0.006, well below the 0.2 level considered a "small" effect. Adverse effects were not systematically assessed or reported. Though Lester et al. argued for the importance of this small effect size when summed across the entire military population, the IoM panel essentially dismissed the results, noting that it did not "find these results meaningful, given the low level of improvement and the very small effect size." Steenkamp, Nash, and Litz (2013) argued that these results are unsurprising, given that a meta-analysis of studies testing the Penn Resiliency

Program on which the Army program was modeled arrived at a similar conclusion (Brunwasser, Gilham, and Kim, 2009).

What constructive lessons regarding ICTs can be learned from the CSF effort?

1. CSF is massive, complex, and multifaceted, and without ICTs the program feasibility and affordability would likely be prohibitive. Without ICTs, high-fidelity administration of CSF is almost certainly impossible.
2. Without an ICT-based assessment platform, the timely and reliable administration of millions of outcome assessments would be cost prohibitive and logistically impossible. While it is difficult to isolate and specifically evaluate this impact of ICT use within CSF, it seems likely that any large-scale universal prevention program will need to use ICTs in a similar way, suggesting that ICTs may enable important new service arrangements.

Alcohol and Substance Misuse

Universal prevention of alcohol misuse, particularly school-based interventions for young people, has been a promising area of research, though controlled trial evidence examining the role of ICTs remains sparse. The potential to generalize school-based programs at the unit level makes these types of programs uniquely appealing for the military context. There is promising early evidence to suggest that school-based interventions can be effective (e.g., Foxcroft and Tsertsvadze, 2011). However, few ICT-related randomized trials have been completed to date.

One example worthy of highlight is a school-based online universal prevention program developed in Australia for cannabis and alcohol. This program, called Climate Schools (Teesson et al., 2014), has been shown in a large randomized trial to lead to improved outcomes at 6- and 12-month follow-up (improvements in alcohol and cannabis knowledge, reduction in average weekly alcohol consumption, reduction in frequency of drinking to excess). The program was also accepted by teachers and students as a means of delivering drug education in schools (Newton et al., 2010) and showed reductions in risk factors associated with substance use in adolescents (Newton et al., 2014a). Preparations are now under way for controlled trial testing in the United Kingdom (Newton et al., 2014b).

In general, randomized trials of computer-based prevention targeting substances other than alcohol appear promising, though perhaps not easily applied in a military context in which these drugs are illegal and likely to lead to initiation of separation proceedings rather than treatment. Wood et al. (2014) conducted a systematic review to examine evidence from programs to prevent substance misuse. A comprehensive search of eight literature databases identified three randomized trials evaluating computer-based programs to prevent or reduce use of drugs. These studies used a variety of intervention approaches, target groups, and settings. The studies found that universal drug prevention programs were effective in reducing the frequency of recreational drug use after 12 months but were not effective immediately after the intervention.

Intimate Partner Relationship Problems

We were unable to identify empirical tests of ICTs designed for universal preventive interventions addressing general intimate partner relationship problems, such as marital quality or satisfaction with intimate partner relationships. However, there are studies of universal prevention for intimate partner violence (IPV), including one randomized preventive intervention trial. Braithwaite and Fincham (2014) completed this trial, comparing a computer-based IPV intervention called ePREP to an active relationship education program for married couples in the community. ePREP intervention reduced physical and psychological aggression among the couples (a 90-percent reduction in expected counts of physical aggression and a modest reduction in self-reported psychological aggression), and these gains were maintained at a one-year follow-up assessment. This approach deserves further study and may offer an ICT-based universal prevention opportunity to reduce interpersonal violence among intimate partners when one or more individuals are serving in the military.

Targeted Prevention

Where universal prevention covers the entire population, *targeted prevention* focuses intervention on a particular subgroup of the population that is at increased risk for a condition. This type of prevention is also referred to as *indicated prevention*, meaning that the prevention is indicated by the subgroup's elevated risk (e.g., people with a history of depression are at increased risk of future depression). A second reason to narrow the target is because an especially good intervention context exists. This *selective prevention* may involve primary care or certain workplace settings. For example, visiting primary care or working in a grocery store may not be a health risk factor, but these settings can present opportunities for preventive screening and referral based on identified risk.

This section on the use of ICTs for targeted prevention will focus on targeted prevention programs that target subgroups at increased risk for adverse mental or behavioral health outcomes. Selective prevention, particularly that completed in health care settings or relying on screening with referral to health care, is addressed in the chapter on treatment. Table 2.1 offers some targeted prevention examples and the risk group and preventive goal potentially associated with each.

Table 2.1. Hypothetical Examples of Targeted Prevention

Risk Group	Intervention	Preventive Goal
Family history of depression	Online depression education	Early treatment-seeking
Recent traumatic event	Online therapy	Reducing the onset or severity of PTSS
Past victim of domestic violence	Online education and assistance resources	Reduced risk of future events
Past citation for driving under influence of alcohol	Online risk education	Prevention of alcohol-related accidents and emergencies
Wounded warrior caregiver	Online caregiver support	Reduction in caregiver depression, anxiety, and absenteeism

Targeted Prevention Applications for Specific Problems

Depression

Muñoz and colleagues have argued that the most feasible and resource efficient prevention programs for depression are those that target groups at relatively high risk for depression over the short term (Muñoz et al., 2010). Among the preventive interventions they highlighted as most promising are Internet-based therapeutic interventions, noting that there is "no reason to assume that they cannot be used as [targeted] preventive interventions" (Muñoz et al., 2010, p. 194). Among the preventive risk groups they identified as important targets are adolescents, postpartum women, persons with physical health conditions, caregivers, and those with subthreshold depression symptoms.

These depression risk groups are relevant to targeted prevention of depression in the military. Adolescents comprise a large proportion of the Air Force. Late adolescence extends to 22 years of age, and in 2012, about 44 percent of active-duty enlisted airmen were 25 years old or less (DoD, 2013). Most military families have one or more members within the biological reproductive ages of roughly 15 to 49 years old, making the postpartum phase very common among military families. Many military families are likely to be caregivers for disabled children or other family members, friends, and "wounded warriors," and some military units (e.g., Warrior Transition Units) are composed of service members benefiting from family and other caregivers.

Another military-relevant target site for preventive work is the workplace. Dietrich et al. (2012) completed a systematic review of preventive workplace interventions for depression. This review sought studies of any preventive workplace interventions for depression, not specifically ICTs. The literature was searched through 2010, identifying 9,173 potential studies of workplace preventive strategies targeting depression. Only one study met their criteria for inclusion (Godard et al., 2006), and that study was not randomized, nor did it assess an ICT-based approach. The importance of this as an area for future military-specific ICT research is obvious.

There is some evidence that Internet-based behavioral programs targeting people with insomnia could offer promise for depression. Ritterband and colleagues (2009) recruited participants through non–health-care-based outreach and then randomized eligible participants to a nine-week structured behavioral Internet intervention for insomnia called SHUTi (Sleep Healthy Using the Internet, 2013) or a control condition. Participants in the SHUTi program experienced large improvements in sleep-related outcomes compared to those receiving the control condition—improvements that were sustained at six-month follow-up. Subsequent analyses found improvements in associated mental health symptoms and quality of life (Thorndike et al., 2013).

Generally speaking, the empirical evidence for non–health-care-based targeted preventive interventions for depression remains unclear, despite the theoretical promise of this strategy. It is likely that this strategy will continue to be an active area of intervention development and experimental research in the future.

Posttraumatic Stress Symptoms

There has been considerable debate around the role of targeted posttraumatic stressor prevention measures. A convincing scientific literature now exists to suggest that early psychological debriefing (a strategy in which all individuals exposed to a traumatic event are provided individual or group psychotherapy designed to prevent subsequent psychological sequelae) is ineffective at best (Roberts et al., 2009). In some well-designed randomized trials, individuals who received early psychological interventions suffered *worse* outcomes than individuals who did not (Mayou, Ehlers, and Hobbs, 2000). These experimental findings suggest that an intense focus on traumatic events within days of the trauma may contribute to future psychological symptoms. It is unclear at this time what psychological help, if any, should be offered in the aftermath of traumatic events. Therefore, this is not a promising area for the mental health use of ICTs.

Alcohol and Substance Misuse

Alcohol is a major factor in IPV (Foran and O'Leary, 2008) and preventable fatal injuries, including suicide (Smith, Branas, and Miller, 1999). There are reasons to suspect that serious military career consequences may result in underreporting of alcohol misuse on routine screening (Santiago et al., 2010), yet studies suggest it may be the most common military behavioral health problem (Messer et al., 2004; Santiago et al., 2010). The use of single-session personalized feedback interventions without specific therapeutic guidance has been well studied in student and general populations (Riper et al., 2009). These interventions are feasible and offer a potentially cost-effective way of reducing hazardous drinking that may offer important utility in the military context. The Internet offers ample opportunities to deliver personalized feedback interventions on a broad scale, and problem drinkers find Internet-based interventions acceptable (Riper et al., 2009).

Related to personalized feedback interventions are "social norms" interventions, which aim to reduce misperceptions among youths who participate in hazardous drinking regarding how their peers drink. One meta-analysis of social norms interventions for alcohol misuse found that web-based interventions were comparable to individual face-to-face methods and that both were "probably effective" in the short term. The authors speculated that web-based feedback probably offers a more favorable cost-to-benefit ratio for use as a targeted prevention measure (Moreira, Smith, and Foxcroft, 2009).

A meta-analysis of computer-based approaches for alcohol and tobacco use led to an effect size of 0.2 for alcohol misuse and 0.14 for tobacco cessation (Rooke et al., 2010). These are small but potentially important effect sizes for use as a large-scale targeted preventive measure. This meta-analysis, which reviewed 42 effect sizes obtained from 34 studies involving 10,632 participants, found that the level of therapist involvement did not predict treatment outcome, with studies involving minimal contact producing larger effect sizes than studies involving higher levels of contact. This finding is in contrast to the evidence pertaining to computer-based interventions for depression and anxiety; therapist contact with computer-based interventions for those conditions leads to better outcomes and adherence (Richards and Richardson, 2012). Finally, the study by Rooke et al. (2010) found no significant outcome differences in relation to treatment location, provision of normative feedback, availability of a discussion feature, inclusion of entertainment features, number of treatment sessions, or emphasis on relapse prevention.

On the whole, targeted preventive measures using the Internet for at-risk drinkers appear to represent a promising ICT direction, though the evidence remains somewhat mixed.

Intimate Partner Relationship Problems

There is considerable interest in addressing the relationship of mental health problems and substance use with relationship difficulties, and intimate partner violence (IPV) in particular. Victims of IPV, particularly women victims, are at about double the risk for new onset of depressive symptoms, suicide attempts, and substance misuse compared to the general population (Devries et al., 2013). Furthermore, depressive symptoms among women are related to subsequent IPV (Devries et al., 2013). To prevent and reduce depression and associated sequelae, continued research is needed that evaluates IPV prevention strategies (Beydoun et al., 2012). One meta-analysis showed improvements in substance misuse among women with a history of IPV who received preventive services (Fowler and Falkner, 2011). While the role of ICTs in prevention targeted to victims of IPV is less than clear, these findings, combined with the earlier findings suggesting that ICTs can help deliver universal prevention of IPV, make this strategy a particularly interesting area for future ICT application and program testing and development.

Behavioral Health Prevention Opportunities

The existing evidence regarding both universal and targeted preventive interventions to reduce depression, PTSS, alcohol and substance misuse, and relationship problems is weak in two ways:

1. There is little evidence for positive effects of interventions that adopt these strategies.
2. Since few interventions have been tested experimentally, there is little evidence, either positive or negative, of the many potential interventions that could use these strategies. Moreover, the costs and potential harms of these interventions have generally not been investigated.

What are the implications that this body of evidence has for the future of ICT applications in mental health?

1. Data suggest that military resilience programs that target reductions in deployment-related PTSS have made little impact, particularly when compared to the resources required to deliver them. There is no data to inform concerns that these programs may raise mental health stigma.
2. Use of the Internet, computers, and smartphones for mental health education is important. Cautious expansion of educational approaches using increasingly ubiquitous tools seems reasonable, though evidence from rigorous studies is currently lacking.
3. Several examples from school settings and the school-based prevention literature may present interesting analogies to the military and unit-based prevention efforts. These analogies may afford opportunities to translate evidence from universal preventive research in the general population into real-world military adaptation and use. It is not surprising that young military men and women face many challenges that are typical of civilians in their age group, including adolescent patterns of substance use, emotional distress, exposure to traumatic events, and relationship problems.
4. Efforts to implement ICT-based universal preventive interventions might prioritize the problems of alcohol misuse and IPV. Universal prevention of depression, anxiety, and PTSS appears unlikely to offer easy gains or major dividends in the near term, and the risk is greater that resources programmed toward these latter problems will be resources lost.

3. ICTs in the Clinical Process

In this chapter, we move from the application of ICTs to preclinical public health interventions to their application in the clinical process itself. For analytic purposes, we divide the clinical process into four stages of care that occur after an individual has been referred to a clinician, either for a particular condition that has been identified through screening or for general preventive care. The distinction between prevention, discussed in the previous chapter, and the clinical process, described here, is that the stages described here presume that an individual has come into contact with a clinical care provider.

In the Waiting Room: Patient Education and Activation

Interventions have been developed to target the time period between an individual's referral to treatment and her or his initial face-to-face interaction with a provider. For instance, it is common for patients to complete checklists of their medical history, their current health status, or their health behaviors while they sit in the waiting room to see a clinician or at home prior to an appointment (Fann et al., 2009; Kobak et al., 1997). This information is then passed to the clinician, who can then be more efficient by focusing on specific issues of concern. With respect to behavioral health, patients may be asked to complete standard screening instruments for depression (Kim et al., 2011), relationship problems, suicidality, or substance misuse. Interventions during this stage aim to orient the patient to his or her health and health care and facilitate interaction with the provider, particularly when the actual time that a patient spends in face-to-face interaction with a provider is very brief.

A number of potential applications of ICTs during the preclinical phase have been described in the literature, although actual testing of these applications is quite limited (Fann et al., 2009; Lawrence et al., 2010; Kim et al., 2011). Some applications are as simple as filling out a standard checklist using a secure smartphone app or website, which automatically transmits the data to the provider's office in advance of the appointment (Fann et al., 2009). More sophisticated applications could use the unique features of the smartphone to collect data that would otherwise be very difficult to collect, such as multiple assessments taken over time that would provide more detailed and clinically relevant information. For instance, patients concerned with insomnia could record their sleep habits (actively or passively) for a period of time prior to the appointment.

Behavioral health interventions during the preclinical period have received particular attention because of the concern that many patients may be reluctant to discuss behavioral health problems with their clinicians. In fact, there is concern among researchers that simply filling out a screening instrument and sharing the results with the provider may not be sufficient to overcome to barriers to help-seeking for such stigmatized problems as depression. To improve the likelihood that patients will discuss behavioral health problems with their health care providers, interventions that focus on "patient activation" or "patient engagement," a combination of psycho-education and coaching, have been developed. These programs aim to empower patients as advocates for their own care by providing information on clinical options tailored to their current health status (Bell et al., 2010). For instance, Kravitz et al. (2013) tested an interactive multimedia computer program (IMCP) that integrated a screening instrument for depression with psychoeducational content tailored to the individuals' screening results. The IMCP was provided to patients in the waiting room prior to a visit with a primary care clinician. Depressed patients who received the IMCP were more likely to receive a medication consultation or a referral to mental health specialty care than were control patients.

In the Doctor's Office: Enhancing the Clinical Encounter

The next phase in the clinical process is the actual interaction between the clinician and the patient. ICT applications in this phase fall into three categories:

- clinical decision support
- telemedicine
- ICT-based treatments.

Each of these applications takes advantage of different information technologies that have become common in medicine, and each has distinctive goals:

- Clinical decision support tools make use of electronic health records to provide clinicians with information to assist in diagnosis or treatment. The health records can integrate information across time and across multiple providers, which makes them particularly useful for patients with complex medical needs that include behavioral health conditions.
- Telemedicine uses videoconferencing technology to allow clinicians to examine and even treat patients remotely. Methods for delivering behavioral health care via telemedicine have been in use for several decades, and new methods, making use of new technologies, are being continuously introduced.
- ICTs using smartphones or other Internet-connected devices have also been developed to provide treatment directly to patients, potentially obviating the need for a face-to-face encounter with a provider altogether.

In this section we review recent literature on each of these approaches.

Decision Support

Computerized clinical decision support (CCDS) systems are methods for using electronically stored health information, primarily patients' medical records, to provide information to clinicians that will enhance their ability to make evidence-based clinical decisions (Musen, Middleton, and Greenes, 2014). Their goal is to utilize information to improve the quality and efficiency of clinical care. For instance, CCDS systems have been studied and used to assist clinicians with diagnosis, identify potential drug–drug interactions (Wright et al., 2012), remind clinicians to address particular issues (Romano and Stafford, 2011), and provide treatment checklists (Cannon and Allen, 2000). Despite the initial promise that these computerized systems appeared to offer, evidence gathered from research over the past 30 years has been mixed. Reviews of studies of CCDS systems have generally found evidence of positive effects on some clinical process outcomes, such as improvements in screening rates, but little evidence of positive effects on patient outcomes (Garg et al., 2005; Bright et al., 2012; Jaspers et al., 2011; Damiani et al., 2010; Wears and Berg, 2005). In particular, CCDS systems appear to have the most positive impact in clinical settings where the amount of information on which decisions are based is small, such as drug ordering or preventive care reminders (Jaspers et al., 2011).

Within mental health, there has been extensive interest in applying CCDS systems in a number of arenas, including care for complex patients with comorbid physical and mental health conditions (Woltmann et al., 2011), child psychiatry (Co et al., 2010), and treatment of common mental health conditions in primary care settings (Rollman et al., 2002). Evidence that these systems can, on their own, improve outcomes for treatment of mental health conditions in primary care is weak (Gilbody et al., 2003). For instance, one of the earliest trials of this approach examined a system that used an electronic health record to provide feedback and treatment advice on depression treatment to primary care clinicians. Patients who screened positive for depression and were randomized to this intervention were not more likely to receive guideline-concordant care or have better depression outcomes than similar patients randomized to usual care (Rollman et al., 2002). However, CCDS systems have played important roles as components of comprehensive behavioral health care models for primary care (Powell et al., 2012). For instance, the IMPACT model, which has been shown to improve depression outcomes for older adults by providing care management in primary care clinics (Unützer et al., 2002b), makes use of a web-based decision support system (Unützer et al., 2002a).

CCDS systems have also been developed to promote the use of brief interventions for alcohol misuse. Brief interventions aim to alter the course of alcohol misuse by providing focused counseling to patients at high risk for alcohol-related problems, frequently in an emergency room following an alcohol-related medical emergency. Studies have found that brief interventions, usually counseling sessions in which a clinician discusses the potential long-term consequence of alcohol misuse, are effective in reducing long-term alcohol misuse trajectories (Bien, Miller, and Tonigan, 1993). An RCT conducted in the U.S. Department of Veterans Affairs (VA) system found that use of brief interventions increased significantly when an electronic clinical reminder to provide them was introduced into the electronic health record (Lapham et al., 2012).

Another potentially important innovation that aims to improve clinical decisionmaking through information technology is the integration of electronic health records through a health information exchange (HIE). The need for an HIE grows out of fragmentation within the health care system that creates barriers to the exchange of information between providers. For instance, historically, no medical information has been shared between the DoD and VA health systems, so that clinicians seeing patients in the VA system had no direct access to the medical records on their patients covering their time in active-duty service. A new HIE system called the Virtual Lifetime Electronic Record, which combines DoD and VA medical records into a single system, is currently being deployed across the VA system (Byrne et al., 2014).

Telemedicine

Telemedicine has been used to provide mental health care (i.e., telemental health care) remotely for well over 50 years (Hilty et al., 2013) and is currently in use routinely in some military health settings. Research has demonstrated that care provided by video link is equally as effective as care provided in person and that it is acceptable to both clinicians and patients. The American Telemedicine Association (Yellowlees et al., 2010; Turvey et al., 2013) and the American Association of Child and Adolescent Psychiatry (Myers et al., 2008) have developed guidelines for telemental health. With respect to specific disorders, studies have found telemedicine to be effective in providing care for depression (Fortney et al., 2013; Fortney et al., 2007; Ruskin et al., 2004; Moreno et al., 2012), PTSD (Frueh et al., 2007; Morland et al., 2010; Germain et al., 2009), and substance misuse (Frueh, Henderson, and Myrick, 2005). Given the extensive literature on telehealth and its current use in the Air Force (Swigert et al., 2014; Woodson, 2014), we focus here on two recent extensions of telemental health practice: smartphone-based videoconferencing and online chat.

The video capacity of smartphones allows for remote face-to-face contact between clinicians and patients, which could be used to provide or support mental health treatment (Chan et al., 2014). The increasing sophistication of free smartphone apps, including assurance that they meet federal government standards for secure transmission of protected health information, promises to make these methods more widely used in the future. While there is no reliable information on the extent to which smartphones are currently being used for this purpose, many private psychotherapists advertise their ability to provide care via smartphone. In addition, the nonprofit organization Give an Hour, which connects service members and veterans with free mental health care, offers services using Google Hangouts, a popular, free smartphone video conferencing app.

Online chat, or, more specifically, individual synchronous online chat counseling and therapy, has also become widely available in recent years through numerous online-based private-sector providers (Dowling and Rickwood, 2013). While online chat provides convenience and privacy because it can be used almost anywhere, research evidence concerning the therapeutic efficacy of chat is very scarce. A review published in 2013 found only six studies assessing the efficacy of chat. Although the results demonstrate the feasibility of online chat as a therapeutic modality, none of the studies make strong comparisons (e.g., with randomization to intervention and control conditions) between therapy delivered by chat and therapy delivered by other methods (Dowling and Rickwood, 2013). Potential risks to confidentiality of treatment that is not face to face and that may be stored without participant knowledge on an Internet device should also be considered.

ICT-Based Treatments

ICTs are also being developed as the primary modality of behavioral health treatments. These ICTs may involve some interaction with a clinician, but the clinician's role is clearly supplemental to the ICT itself, through which the primary treatment is administered. In fact, the first computerized behavioral health treatments were developed in the 1980s and 1990s, prior to broad access to the Internet, and some of the current leaders in this area are updated versions of those original computer-based programs that now take advantage of current technologies (Pelosi and Lewis, 1989). The programs utilize technology in combination with traditional face-to-face treatment in a number of different strategies; some involve virtually no clinician input, some involve clinicians at the start of treatment, and some require clinicians to provide substantive feedback, in real time or asynchronously through email, as part of the treatment process (Richards and Richardson, 2012; Barak et al., 2008).

These ICTs promise several distinct advantages over traditional face-to-face treatments. First, they dramatically reduce the need for professional time, thereby reducing the cost of providing care. Second, since the interaction with the clinician is also electronic, usually through text or email, ICTs dramatically expand the geographic reach of treatment systems. ICTs may be particularly valuable in rural or remote areas where treatment infrastructure does not exist. Third, ICTs make treatment more convenient by removing the need for appointments and the need for the provider and patient to be together at any particular point in time.

At the same time, ICT behavioral health treatments also face a number of challenges, some of which are shared by traditional face-to-face treatments. Most important among these is treatment dropout. Evidence suggests that when ICTs are provided to a general population, their uptake is low, and most people who begin a course of ICT treatment do not continue long enough to receive clinical benefit (Christensen, Griffiths, and Farrer, 2009). Adherence to treatment over time may be higher among patients with strong motivations to pursue treatment and may be improved through further technological enhancements to the treatment programs, such as reminders, incentives, or direct clinician involvement.

Most Internet-based treatments that have been developed and tested scientifically are based on cognitive behavioral therapy (CBT). Traditional face-to-face CBT is the most intensively studied psychotherapy, and it has been found to be effective in treating anxiety and depressive syndromes and a broad variety of related syndromes in hundreds of randomized clinical trials (Hofmann et al., 2012; Hunsley, Elliott, and Therrien, 2014). For instance, a review conducted in 2012 found 269 meta-analytic studies of CBT published since 2000 (Hofmann et al., 2012). The most commonly studied applications were to anxiety and depressive disorders, but meta-analyses have also been conducted to assess the efficacy of CBT for substance use disorders, schizophrenia and other psychotic disorders, bipolar disorder, eating disorders, insomnia, personality disorders, anger and aggression, criminal behaviors, general stress, distress due to medical conditions, chronic pain, and chronic fatigue (Hofmann et al., 2012). CBT aims to alleviate psychological symptoms by teaching patients skills that enable them to avoid maladaptive cognitions. Internet CBT (iCBT) teaches the skills taught in traditional CBT through a mix of informational slides and videos accessible over the Internet (Hedman et al., 2011).

A course of iCBT consists of online classes or self-administered sessions, typically fewer in number than would generally be expected in a course of traditional CBT. The many iCBT programs that have been developed vary with respect to a number of important design factors. Most importantly, they vary in the extent to which a clinician is involved in the treatment. Some iCBT programs are completely self-guided, meaning that there is no clinician input into the treatment process. Others involve minimal clinician involvement, often at the beginning of the treatment to provide screening and orientation, and others involve more extensive clinician involvement throughout the treatment, usually providing feedback to patients on their homework assignments. Clinician feedback is generally provided via email, although some programs include real-time communication between patients and clinicians (Richards and Richardson, 2012). To date, iCBT has been tested in clinical trials to treat depression, panic disorder, social phobia, PTSD, generalized anxiety disorder, obsessive-compulsive disorder, eating disorders, health anxiety, chronic pain, tinnitus, irritable bowel syndrome, sexual dysfunction, cannabis use, nicotine addiction, pathological gambling, and nonspecific distress (Hedman et al., 2011).

Findings from RCTs of iCBT have generally been favorable. Richards and Richardson (2012) conducted a meta-analysis of 19 RCTs of iCBT treatment for depression and found that, on average, the treatments reduced depressive symptoms by over half a standard deviation, an effect considered moderate in size (effect size $d = 0.56$, $p < 0.001$) (Richards and Richardson, 2012). In this study, the estimated impact of iCBT was larger for those programs that involved clinicians in the treatment process (effect size $d = 0.78$) than for those with no provider support (effect size $d = 0.36$). Hedman et al. (2011) reviewed iCBT treatments for a broader range of clinical syndromes and found large positive effects for treatment of depression, anxiety disorders, severe health anxiety, irritable bowel disorder, female sexual dysfunction, eating disorders, cannabis use, and pathological gambling. Smaller positive treatment effects were found for a range of other clinical applications.

Studies that have compared iCBT with traditional CBT have generally found similar positive effects on clinical outcomes. Hedman et al. (2012) reviewed 12 RCTs that compared the effects of these two treatment modalities and found no significant difference between them (Hedman et al., 2011). The same finding was reported in another review (Andrews et al., 2010). However, there is good reason to be cautious about this particular finding. Studies may have small sample sizes that prevent well-powered comparisons of treatment effects between these two treatment modalities. In addition, given the variation in treatment effects within iCBTs based on the extent of clinician involvement (Richards and Richardson, 2012), it is likely that face-to-face CBT may be more effective than many types of iCBT against which it has not been directly compared in the literature. A review by Newman et al. (2011) suggests that iCBT with low involvement of clinicians may be more appropriate for motivated patients with anxiety disorders, while iCBT or face-to-face CBT may be more appropriate for patients with lower motivation or more serious disorders, including depression.

We include a further cautionary note regarding attrition from web-based treatment programs, including iCBT. In clinical trials, attrition from iCBT is similar to that from in-person CBT (van Ballegooijen et al., 2014). However, clinical trials are likely to include highly motivated patients who have sought and made contact with medical treatment and research teams that work hard to keep patients in treatment over time. If the target population of Internet programs includes individuals who would not otherwise have access to treatment, then they are not well represented by these samples. The problem of attrition from Internet-based treatments has been widely recognized in the literature (Christensen and Mackinnon, 2006; Eysenbach, 2005), particularly for programs that are simply made available online without clinician involvement (Christensen, Griffiths, and Farrer, 2009; Kelders et al., 2012).

In Treatment: Improving Adherence to Treatment

One of the most important areas of ICT development in medicine has been in applications that supplement, rather than replace, existing in-person treatments using smartphones and other Internet-based technologies (Clough and Casey, 2011b; Clough and Casey, 2011a; Boschen and Casey, 2008). These approaches make use of the unique values of both face-to-face interaction with a clinician and frequent information exchange using ubiquitous technology at the same time. Treatment adherence, defined as "the extent to which a patient acts in accordance with the prescribed interval, and dose of a dosing regimen" (Dayer et al., 2013, p. 172), is a primary target in this area. This type of application is particularly relevant for behavioral health because of the very high level of dropout from traditional treatments and because of the need for patients to be continuously engaged in their treatment over an extended period of time to achieve positive clinical results.

Medication Adherence

Across health conditions, the proportion of patients who adhere to medication regimens is about 50 percent (Haynes, McDonald, and Garg, 2002). Designers of smartphone applications have focused on developing apps to remind people to take their medication; a review of app marketplaces conducted in August and September 2012 found 147 distinct apps for medication reminders (Dayer et al., 2013). There is strong evidence that these apps are acceptable to patient populations (Miller and Himelhoch, 2013) and to clinicians (Kuhn et al., 2014). However, there remains a great deal of uncertainty regarding the extent to which the apps would be used, even when offered. For instance, in a study of a medication reminder app offered by a health system to its enrollees, fewer than 30 percent of individuals who downloaded the app and agreed to have their use of it monitored used the app at least once a week for four weeks or more (Becker et al., 2013). Moreover, use was more common among older patients with severe medical conditions, such as cancer, heart disease, or a history of organ transplant, than among younger, healthier patients similar to the Air Force population.

Adherence to Psychological Treatments

While medication reminders are a straightforward and relatively simple function for smartphone apps to fill, there are also many attempts to apply ICTs as adjuncts to more complex psychological treatments (Boschen and Casey, 2008; Robertson et al., 2006). These ICT applications aim to improve adherence to treatment by maintaining communication between patient and therapist between sessions—e.g., using text messages or email (Aguilera and Muñoz, 2011; Murdoch and Connor-Greene, 2000)—and enabling patients to complete therapeutic homework assignments with a phone or computer so that they were transmitted directly to their therapists (Clough and Casey, 2011b; Clough and Casey, 2011a).

In many regards, these ICTs are natural extensions of established, evidence-based practices that have contributed to considerable advances in convenience for both patients and therapists. Both patients and therapists report high levels of comfort using them and are more likely to find them acceptable than online treatments. For instance, a study of marriage and family therapists found that while about three-fourths felt very uncomfortable using the Internet as the primary mode of treatment, only about one-fourth felt very uncomfortable with the Internet as a supplement to in-person treatment (Hertlein, Blumer, and Smith, 2014). In a pilot study of patients with PTSD, the large majority were comfortable with monitoring of symptom change over time after hospitalization via text message (Price et al., 2014). In the RAND survey of airmen mentioned at the beginning of Chapter 1, 46 percent of airmen reported using ICTs to access mental health information (Miller et al., 2014).

Research on the effectiveness of treatment adherence apps suggests some promising effects, but more research is needed to develop strategies for specific disorders and populations. A systematic review conducted in 2013 found 59 clinical trials of mobile technologies to improve chronic disease management. However, only four of these trials met high standards of evidence for treatment efficacy, including a low risk of bias in the results (Free et al., 2013). The main focus of the high-quality clinical trials was in patients with very serious illnesses—e.g., management of HIV disease and post-transplant health status, and the tested apps showed positive effects. However, this evidence should also be considered against some negative evidence. A recent clinical trial that aimed to improve adherence to psychotherapy found that texted appointment reminders had no effect on whether patients showed up for their appointments (Clough and Casey, 2014).

Maintaining Treatment Gains over Time

It can be challenging to maintain gains made in treatment over the long term. ICTs provide a means for delivering supplemental treatments after formal treatment has ended (Clough and Casey, 2011b; Price et al., 2013). These approaches are generally at a low level of intensity with minor involvement of clinicians. However, they may be sufficient to help former patients maintain their well-being and avoid relapse of acute illness. Studies have examined online chat groups (Golkaramnay et al., 2007), text and phone support (S. Bauer et al., 2012; Robinson et al., 2006), and phone-based monitoring (McKay et al., 2010) to address a range of moderate to severe mental health problems. None of these approaches have been tested in randomized trials, but acceptability and adherence have been high. Interventions in this category have tended to focus on patients with serious psychopathology, such as patients being discharged from inpatient treatment, patients with eating disorders, and patients with alcohol dependence.

Clinical Opportunities for Behavioral Health

Many ICT applications have been proposed, and many are currently being developed. This is a fast-moving area of technology development, and the research that can provide direction is not keeping up with the pace of change. But it is an area in which mental health providers need to stay apprised of advancements, as we expect continuing developments. Though there is a large literature, the literature includes a very high proportion of descriptive papers, reviews, and non-controlled studies, so conclusions are hard to draw. For instance, the review of smartphone apps for mental health care by Donker et al. (2013) started with over 5,000 abstracts and found only eight controlled studies, and most of those were of low quality. Most studies with controls are of low quality because they do not randomize individuals to treatments, a crucial methodological consideration when judging the validity of study findings. Also, program developers often conduct these studies and have a clear interest in their success. There is a high likelihood that negative studies are not published ("file drawer bias"). The weak state of the scientific evidence despite the seemingly large size of the related literature has been noted in recent publications (Tomlinson et al., 2013).

The lack of solid research evidence to date should not be mistaken, however, for a lack of promise for the Air Force. ICTs provide an obvious advance in convenience for both providers and clinicians in certain common situations in which they carry very low risk. The frequent moves and inflexible schedules of Air Force personnel may make these features of ICTs particularly valuable in the Air Force context. In particular, simple but reliable methods for patient-clinician communication between therapy sessions appear to be a promising avenue. Similarly, the established value of iCBT may have a clear role to play in the Air Force context. While there may be no off-the-shelf products that the Air Force can simply purchase and implement, the successes in these areas demonstrated in the literature suggest that they should be priority targets for Air Force efforts.

A persistent issue with technology development and research on ICT applications is the granular level of ICT innovations. ICTs tend to be developed to address needs that arise within particular health systems and for specific target populations. Success may not translate to the military health systems or to the priority Air Force mental health problems. For this reason, development of a strategy for ICTs should start with a detailed understanding of the intended target use. For instance, uptake of an ICT may be very low when considered as a proportion of the entire Air Force population. However, if effectively targeted to a population in need, such as Air Force personnel who change station while in treatment for depression, then even very low uptake may be justified.

Finally, mental health care occurs as part of a complex health system and within a complex military context, both of which include many moving parts. While the incremental advances in convenience provided by ICTs may not register in research studies as improvements in clinical outcomes, their positive impact on treatment processes may represent valuable contributions to the treatment system.

4. Conclusions and Recommendations

ICTs offer a wide range of promising innovative modalities for improving mental health care, but the research evidence regarding their effectiveness is limited with respect to most of the proposed applications of ICTs and the extent to which the evidence that does exist is generalizable to the Air Force population and context. Therefore, a cautious approach to adoption and implementation in the Air Force is recommended because of concerns for efficient use of resources, as well as the safety and privacy of airmen. Although the existing literature is large, few publications bring empirical evidence to bear. As a result, there are few replicated results in the areas of greatest potential Air Force impact or concern. While a primary concern of the Air Force lies in ICT applications that extend the reach of mental health services to airmen who would not otherwise have access to care, evidence in the scientific literature on universal and targeted prevention programs using ICTs is extremely limited. Existing studies are limited by lack of reporting of costs and adverse events, marked intervention heterogeneity, and inconsistent results. The best-studied areas involve the use of ICTs to improve services to *persons already in clinical treatment,* a clinically significant but small population subgroup.

Constructive lessons and opportunities emerge from the available literature, however, and in this chapter we suggest responsible strategies and domains for evidence-informed implementation of behavioral health ICTs in the Air Force. Our recommendations in this regard emphasize precision over speed—successive, incremental gains and a program of measurement-based implementation and process and outcomes monitoring rather than urgent dissemination. The intended result is small but regular gains in efficiency, effectiveness, safety, and reach of preventive and clinical mental health services to airmen and their families.

Answers to Research Questions

This literature review was motivated by four research questions stated in the introductory chapter. Prior to offering recommendations based on the overall literature review, we address each of those questions below:

1. **Can mental health care providers use ICTs to improve the quality and effectiveness of the care they provide to their patients?**

Although the use of ICTs to enhance mental health treatments is frequently mentioned in the literature, we did not find empirical studies that demonstrate positive effects of ICT use on quality or effectiveness. However, the lack of studies in this area should not be interpreted as negative evidence. At this stage in the rapid development of clinical technology, there are many new ways that ICTs can be used to supplement the traditional in-person clinical process, including recording of homework, appointment reminders, access to crisis intervention, and monitoring of sleep, but these functions have yet to be integrated into robust and testable models of clinical care. Evidence of efficacy of ICT-based treatments, in which treatment is moved entirely to an ICT modality, suggests that the more modest uses of ICTs as supplements to traditional care are feasible and promising.

2. **Are there some types of problems better or equally addressed through ICTs and some that should only be done face to face?**

Research directly comparing in-person treatment to ICT-based treatment has not been conducted for most treatment approaches. The major exception to this rule is ICT-based treatment for depression with CBT, where treatment effects in studies of ICTs are similar to those using in-person treatment. However, whether these results can be maintained in practice with primary care clinical populations remains unknown.

3. **Can ICTs improve patient adherence to mental health treatment?**

Although existing research does not rule out this possibility, there is not strong evidence that existing ICTs have been successful in improving patient adherence to treatment, a long-standing problem in behavioral health. Three specific points are worth mentioning in this regard. First, studies of medication adherence have shown positive effects of ICTs, but the target of this research is very different from the Air Force population. Medication adherence is generally studied in older populations, whose cognitive limitations, social isolation, and complex medical conditions make them quite different from the Air Force population. Second, adherence to iCBT is itself quite problematic, with very high rates of dropout. Stand-alone ICT-based treatments are unlikely to result in greater patient adherence. Third, evidence from studies of clinical reminders suggests that they do not have effects on quality of care. However, there is a gap in the literature with respect to use of ICTs to maintain communication with patients and affect their decisionmaking regarding treatment adherence.

4. **Have care options through ICTs enabled mental health professionals to provide care for individuals who otherwise would not have been willing to obtain face-to-face counseling? If so, what do we know about those individuals' demographic characteristics, diagnoses, and hurdles to receiving face-to-face care?**

Telemedicine and ICT-based treatments provide an alternative modality for behavioral health care to individuals who would otherwise not have access to care, particularly those in rural or remote areas. However, critical information on the impact that ICTs can have in expanding utilization of behavioral health treatments is lacking. While promising, some caution is warranted because of low uptake of treatments. Impacts of ICTs on treatment utilization should be closely monitored over time.

General Recommendations

1. **The Air Force should develop and adopt a coordinated interdisciplinary strategy for behavioral health ICT implementation.** Just as important as the question of which ICTs should be used and how and where to use them is the strategy employed for managing emerging health technologies. An Air Force strategy should be developed that makes use of an interdisciplinary mix of professionals with behavioral health, public health, information technology, mental health measurement, and health communications expertise. In addition, efforts to externally contract much of the ICT development and Air Force adaptation will likely require special contracting expertise in one or more of these other interdisciplinary domains to ensure that the right requirements are properly articulated, defined, and reassessed over time, in accordance with incremental and evolving Air Force goals.

   An appropriate Air Force strategy will involve specific areas of importance and emphasis, criteria for deciding when a tool meets safety and implementation assessment standards and when it is ready for field implementation, appropriate intervals for reassessing ICT success and safety against previously articulated standards, how and when to field subsequent design or measurement modifications, and when to pull or modify the tool for lack of impact or adequate safety.

2. **The Air Force should develop standards and objectives for adaptation of ICTs to the unique Air Force context and implement a method for determining when the standard has been met before fielding a given ICT.** ICTs will continue to play a highly visible and public role in the health assistance available to airmen and their families. The visibility of this role will only increase over time. For the safety and effectiveness of the tool as tested in nonmilitary settings to generalize to the military context and population, careful field testing and adaptation of an ICT is necessary to reduce unintended organizational and health consequences and maximize benefits for the intended populations and individuals (Weinick et al., 2011).

3. **Air Force behavioral health ICTs should be designed for monitoring aggregate use and intervention outcomes, including adverse or unintended effects.** An advantage of ICTs apart from their potential to improve health and prevent health problems is the potential for transparent, built-in measurement features. An example to date is the assessment tool built into the comprehensive resilience programs that the services have implemented. The Air Force should remain mindful that behavioral health ICTs are medical devices. In a manner consistent with continuous quality improvement programs in the clinical service delivery domain, establishing the ongoing safety and effectiveness of these ICT-based programs of care is necessary for ongoing, responsible use.

ICTs and Behavioral Health Prevention

In most cases, the level of evidence from published and scientifically valid research trials supporting the preventive use of ICTs for depression, anxiety, PTSS, alcohol misuse, and relationship problems is sparse. Moreover, studies that have been completed consistently fall short in the need to assess and report adverse outcomes. Nonetheless, some opportunities exist.

Education efforts are generally seen as a public good, and the demand for efficacy and safety data is low. Accordingly, efforts to use the Internet, smartphone apps, and similar technologies to increase Air Force and family member understanding of mental health issues and reduce the mystery and stigma that surround them are responsible and well advised. These efforts should be considered against the level of resources necessary to sustain them, given that wide implementation of expensive but ineffective technologies represents a public harm, since these resources could in theory be diverted to projects and interventions that offer more clearly defined benefits to the Air Force and to society.

There is little scientific reason at present to recommend more active ICT-supported psychosocial programs of resilience or prevention of PTSS, depression, or anxiety. Existing efforts are resource intensive, and available evidence suggests that they offer no demonstrable benefit; some have suggested that resilience programs in particular may only increase mental health stigma (Smith, 2013; Eidelson, Pilisuk, and Soldz, 2011). The picture is a little more optimistic with regard to universal and targeted prevention of alcohol misuse and IPV. In both of these areas, there is school-based research that supports the effectiveness of preventive programs among in-school adolescents. Given the relative youth of the Air Force population and opportunities to implement school-based interventions at an analogous unit-based level, this is an area for future Air Force adaptation, research, and implementation. Victims of IPV are at risk for depression, anxiety, PTSS, suicide attempts, and alcohol misuse. There may be unique non–health-care-based opportunities to provide airmen and spouse victims of IPV with ICT-based prevention efforts.

Other preventive recommendations follow.

1. **If the Air Force introduces ICTs for prevention, this should be done after careful review of existing ICTs provided to airmen across DoD, the various services, and supporting private organizations to harmonize efforts with existing programs.** There are currently ongoing efforts to develop and use ICTs for preventive purposes at a variety of military (e.g., the National Center for Telehealth and Technology), governmental (e.g., VA, the Substance Abuse and Mental Health Services Administration), and private organizations (e.g., Military OneSource, Give an Hour). The potential to learn lessons from existing efforts is great, and the potential for duplicated effort unless careful review occurs is significant. At present there is apparently no single comprehensive list of either preventive behavioral health programs or current ICTs available or in use that can serve those purposes.
2. **The Air Force should seek and collate aggregate search engine data from Air Force and DoD websites aiming to provide preventive assistance to airmen and their families.** Our preliminary efforts to assess search engine results from various sources within DoD and private organizations suggest that it is challenging for military agencies to obtain timely or ongoing results of search engine searches. Common search terms used can inform Air Force medical leaders of emerging topics of interest to airmen and family members. This information may be used to suggest to Air Force leaders ways of improving their web presence over time (e.g., focusing on new educational topics of

population interest, removing or revising old topics that are no longer relevant). Evidence to support this approach is currently lacking, but efforts in this regard may offer a simple, low-cost, and beneficial way of enhancing web-based information resources for airmen and their families.

3. **The Air Force should not use ICTs for the purpose of targeting traumatized units or individuals for "critical incident stress debriefings" or "psychological debriefings."** Extensive research in this area is clear. These interventions, particularly when compulsory or otherwise mandated, do not prevent PTSS. While, to date, there are no randomized trials that have tested ICTs for prevention of PTSS using a targeted briefing methodology, there is little reason to suspect that available ICTs offer any new way forward in this preventive area.
4. **The Air Force should consider use of ICTs offering Internet-based personalized single-session feedback for airmen at identified risk for alcohol-related incidents (e.g., past alcohol-related Uniform Code of Military Justice violation, infraction for driving under the influence of alcohol).** Given the high prevalence of alcohol misuse and its links to multiple disciplinary and mental health problems, the use of ICTs to expand access to effective targeted prevention programs is a strategic choice. Studies of targeted prevention of alcohol problems using single-session feedback show effectiveness in young adults. The Internet offers low-cost opportunities to deliver this preventive intervention in ways that are potentially inexpensive and accountable and can be monitored for ongoing effectiveness.
5. **The Air Force should consider the use of ICTs for universal and targeted prevention efforts relating to IPV.** Approximately half of airmen are married, and a much larger proportion are involved in intimate partner relationships. At least one universal preventive model, ePREP, has been carefully studied and has been shown to be effective for preventing IPV. Less clear but important are future Air Force efforts to target victims of IPV for interventions that aim to prevent future depression, anxiety, PTSS, and alcohol and other substance misuse. While this remains an experimental way forward, there is some early evidence of the importance of targeted prevention of IPV, and studies to explore the role of ICTs for targeted prevention in victims of IPV would appear well directed.

ICTs and Behavioral Health Treatment Processes

The role of ICTs in the process of clinical care for mental health and substance misuse is rapidly growing. Some of these applications are backed by substantial evidence of efficacy, but research lags behind the pace of innovation. Most of the applications of ICTs have not been investigated using rigorous tests of efficacy. However, the mere absence of positive evidence of efficacy does not imply that these ICTs should be discouraged, particularly if they provide some obvious gain in efficiency or convenience for patients in the context of an already proven treatment, such as CBT. As with some universal prevention efforts, the likelihood of harm is low, and the primary concerns are with the quality of the intervention and with opportunity costs of investing resources in training and technology required to offer the ICT-based intervention.

Given the expectation of continuing rapid change in this area in coming years, one goal of Air Force policy should be to provide some guidance to airmen and their clinicians regarding which of the thousands of ICTs available are of sufficient quality and reliability to warrant use in clinical treatment. In some cases, the Air Force may identify specific ICT-based treatment programs in the interest of consistency across providers. For instance, it may be efficient to choose a single iCBT program that would be used across the Air Force. In other cases, providers may benefit from guidance on a variety of available ICTs from which they might choose to meet the needs of particular patients. For instance, patients may benefit from having a variety of smartphone apps for medication reminders available to them.

As with ICTs for prevention, the development of policies and recommendations for specific ICTs in this domain should involve input from clinicians and patients; consideration of the specific context of the Air Force as it relates to mental health treatment; and close monitoring of uptake, usage, and satisfaction with ICTs over time. In particular, we recommend adoption of ICTs for three specific purposes:

1. **The Air Force should adopt an Internet-based treatment program for depression and anxiety, with tailoring to the Air Force population.** The evidence regarding the efficacy of Internet-based CBT is strong and consistent across multiple studies. An iCBT program could fill an important niche in the mental health care delivery system in the Air Force by providing a treatment option for airmen who are remote from treatment, highly mobile, or concerned about the stigma of attending a mental health clinic. If a decision is made to adopt an iCBT program, the Air Force will need to make several additional decisions regarding the selection of the specific program, the amount of clinician guidance that would be involved, the sites in which it would be recommended (e.g., publicly, in primary care, or in mental health specialty care), and the amount of tailoring to the Air Force population and culture that would be required. This decision should be guided by input from airmen and the clinicians who provide their care. After introducing an iCBT program, its usage, including the number of people who initiate treatment using the program, the completion rates, and satisfaction with the program, should be monitored over time to ensure that the program is reaching the intended population.
2. **The future development of Internet-based treatments for substance misuse should be closely monitored.** At present, the evidence does not suggest that existing off-the-shelf programs are likely to be effective in reducing substance misuse. However, some recent developments that hold promise for military populations, including active-duty service members and Operation Enduring Freedom/Operation Iraqi Freedom veterans, are currently being tested and may prove valuable additions to Air Force treatment offerings. In particular, the most promising programs could enroll patients who have self-identified as having an alcohol use problem and are highly motivated to enter treatment. As with the recommendation for iCBT above, any decision to adopt an Internet-based substance misuse program should be made with input from airmen and their clinicians, adaptation to the Air Force population, and consistent monitoring of usage following implementation.

3. **The Air Force should select smartphone apps that airmen can use to monitor their medication and communicate with mental health clinicians between in-person visits.** For both of these functions, evidence suggests that smartphone apps provide effective tools that make adherence to treatment more convenient. Given the very large number of apps currently available, the selection of specific apps will require an extensive review of existing options.

The rapidly changing field of ICT applications to mental health care promises to improve treatment systems in ways that address long-standing problems in both the civilian and military service systems. However, at this point in time, very few ICT applications have moved from promising to proven technologies. If we apply common standards for evidence-based medical interventions, which would require that interventions be tested by independent research groups in high-quality RCTs, only a small handful of ICTs, notably those designed for iCBT, would receive definitive support. Other ICT applications have not attained this high level of evidence required to demonstrate efficacy but nonetheless appear to be promising based on the convenience and efficiency they add to established evidence-based treatments and evidence of their acceptability to patients and providers. This situation is likely to change as the research literature and clinical experience with ICTs grows and consensus forms on which ICT applications are of greatest benefit to patients.

Bibliography

Aguilera, Adrian, and Ricardo F. Muñoz, "Text Messaging as an Adjunct to CBT in Low-Income Populations: A Usability and Feasibility Pilot Study," *Professional Psychology: Research and Practice*, Vol. 42, No. 6, 2011, pp. 472–478.

Air Combat Command, "Comprehensive Airmen Fitness," undated. As of September 26, 2014: http://www.acc.af.mil/library/comprehensiveairmanfitness/

Andrews, G., P. Cuijpers, M. G. Craske, P. McEvoy, and N. Titov, "Computer Therapy for the Anxiety and Depressive Disorders Is Effective, Acceptable and Practical Health Care: A Meta-Analysis," *PLoS One*, Vol. 5, No. 10, 2010, p. e13196. As of September 26, 2014: http://www.ncbi.nlm.nih.gov/pubmed/20967242

Barak, A., Liat Hen, Meyran Boniel-Nissim, and Na'ama Shapira, "A Comprehensive Review and a Meta-Analysis of the Effectiveness of Internet-Based Psychotherapeutic Interventions," *Journal of Technology in Human Services*, Vol. 26, No. 2/4, 2008, pp. 109–160.

Bauer, A. M., S. M. Thielke, W. Katon, J. Unützer, and P. Arean, "Aligning Health Information Technologies with Effective Service Delivery Models to Improve Chronic Disease Care," *Preventive Medicine*, Vol. 66C, 2014, pp. 167–172.

Bauer, S., E. Okon, R. Meermann, and H. Kordy, "Technology-Enhanced Maintenance of Treatment Gains in Eating Disorders: Efficacy of an Intervention Delivered via Text Messaging," *Journal of Consulting and Clinical Psychology*, Vol. 80, No. 4, August 2012, pp. 700–706. As of September 26, 2014: http://www.ncbi.nlm.nih.gov/pubmed/22545736

Becker, S., A. Kribben, S. Meister, C. J. Diamantidis, N. Unger, and A. Mitchell, "User Profiles of a Smartphone Application to Support Drug Adherence—Experiences from the iNephro Project," *PLoS One*, Vol. 8, No. 10, 2013, p. e78547. As of September 26, 2014: http://www.ncbi.nlm.nih.gov/pubmed/24194946

Bell, R. A., D. A. Paterniti, R. Azari, P. R. Duberstein, R. M. Epstein, A. B. Rochlen, M. D. Johnson, S. E. Orrange, C. Slee, and R. L. Kravitz, "Encouraging Patients with Depressive Symptoms to Seek Care: A Mixed Methods Approach to Message Development," *Patient Education Counseling*, Vol. 78, No. 2, February 2010, pp. 198–205. As of September 26: 2014: http://www.ncbi.nlm.nih.gov/pubmed/19674862

Bennett, G. G., and R. E. Glasgow, "The Delivery of Public Health Interventions via the Internet: Actualizing Their Potential," *Annual Review of Public Health*, Vol. 30, 2009, pp. 273–292.

Beydoun, H. A., M. A. Beydoun, J. S. Kaufman, B. Lo, and A. B. Zonderman, “Intimate Partner Violence Against Adult Women and its Association with Major Depressive Disorder, Depressive Symptoms and Postpartum Depression: A Systematic Review and Meta-Analysis,” *Social Science and Medicine*, Vol. 75, No. 6, September 2012, pp. 959–975. As of September 26: http://www.ncbi.nlm.nih.gov/pubmed/22694991

Bien, T. H., W. R. Miller, and J. S. Tonigan, “Brief Interventions for Alcohol Problems: A Review,” *Addiction*, Vol. 88, No. 3, March 1993, pp. 315–335.

Boschen, Mark J., and Leanne M. Casey, “The Use of Mobile Telephones as Adjuncts to Cognitive Behavioral Psychotherapy,” *Professional Psychology: Research and Practice*, Vol. 39, No. 5, 2008, pp. 546–552.

Braithwaite, S. R., and F. D. Fincham, “Computer-Based Prevention of Intimate Partner Violence in Marriage,” *Behaviour Research and Therapy*, Vol. 54, March 2014, pp. 12–21. As of September 26, 2014: http://www.ncbi.nlm.nih.gov/pubmed/24463577

Bright, T. J., A. Wong, R. Dhurjati, E. Bristow, L. Bastian, R. R. Coeytaux, G. Samsa, V. Hasselblad, J. W. Williams, M. D. Musty, L. Wing, A. S. Kendrick, G. D. Sanders, and D. Lobach, “Effect of Clinical Decision-Support Systems: A Systematic Review,” *Annals of Internal Medicine*, Vol. 157, No. 1, July 3, 2012, pp. 29–43. As of September 26, 2014: http://www.ncbi.nlm.nih.gov/pubmed/22751758

Brunwasser, S. M., J. E. Gillham, and E. S. Kim, “A Meta-Analytic Review of the Penn Resiliency Program’s Effect on Depressive Symptoms,” *Journal of Consulting and Clinical Psychology*, Vol. 77, No. 6, 2009, pp. 1042–1054. As of September 26, 2014: http://www.ncbi.nlm.nih.gov/pubmed/19968381

Byrne, Colene M., Lauren M. Mercincavage, Omar Bouhaddou, Jamie R. Bennett, Eric C. Pan, Nathan E. Botts, Lois M. Olinger, Elaine Hunolt, Karl H. Banty, and Tim Cromwell, “The Department of Veterans Affairs’ (VA) Implementation of the Virtual Lifetime Electronic Record (VLER): Findings and Lessons Learned from Health Information Exchange at 12 Sites," *International Journal of Medical Informatics*, Vol. 83, No. 8, August 2014, pp. 537–547.

Cannon, D. S., and S. N. Allen, “A Comparison of the Effects of Computer and Manual Reminders on Compliance with a Mental Health Clinical Practice Guideline,” *Journal of the American Medical Informatics Association*, Vol. 7, No. 2, March–April 2000, pp. 196–203. As of September 26, 2014: http://www.ncbi.nlm.nih.gov/pubmed/10730603

Chan, Steven Richard, John Torous, Ladson Hinton, and Peter Yellowlees, "Mobile Tele-Mental Health: Increasing Applications and a Move to Hybrid Models of Care," *Healthcare*, Vol. 2, No. 2, 2014, pp. 220–233.

Cheung, Ken, and Naihua Duan, "Design of Implementation Studies for Quality Improvement Programs: An Effectiveness–Cost-Effectiveness Framework," *American Journal of Public Health*, Vol. 104, No. 1, 2014, pp. e23–e30.

Christensen, H., K. M. Griffiths, and L. Farrer, "Adherence in Internet Interventions for Anxiety and Depression," *Journal of Medical Internet Research*, Vol. 11, No. 2, 2009, p. e13. As of September 26, 2014:
http://www.ncbi.nlm.nih.gov/pubmed/19403466

Christensen, H., and A. Mackinnon, "The Law of Attrition Revisited," *Journal of Medical Internet Research*, Vol. 8, No. 3, July–September 2006, p. e20.

Clarke, G., and B. J. Yarborough, "Evaluating the Promise of Health IT to Enhance/Expand the Reach of Mental Health Services," *General Hospital Psychiatry*, Vol. 35, No. 4, 2013, pp. 339–344.

Clough, B. A., and L. M. Casey, "Technological Adjuncts to Enhance Current Psychotherapy Practices: A Review," *Clinical Psychology Review*, Vol. 31, No. 3, April 2011a, pp. 279–292. As of September 26, 2014:
http://www.ncbi.nlm.nih.gov/pubmed/21382535

———, "Technological Adjuncts to Increase Adherence to Therapy: A Review," *Clinical Psychology Review*, Vol. 31, No. 5, July 2011b, pp. 697–710. As of September 26, 2014:
http://www.ncbi.nlm.nih.gov/pubmed/21497153

———, "Using SMS Reminders in Psychology Clinics: A Cautionary Tale," *Behavioural and Cognitive Psychotherapy*, epub February 4, 2014, pp. 1–12. As of September 26, 2014:
http://www.ncbi.nlm.nih.gov/pubmed/24495365

Co, J. P., S. A. Johnson, E. G. Poon, J. Fiskio, S. R. Rao, J. Van Cleave, J. M. Perrin, and T. G. Ferris, "Electronic Health Record Decision Support and Quality of Care for Children with ADHD," *Pediatrics,* Vol. 126, No. 2, August 2010, pp. 239–246. As of September 26, 2014:
http://www.ncbi.nlm.nih.gov/pubmed/20643719

Cornum, R., M. D. Matthews, and M. E. P. Seligman, "Comprehensive Soldier Fitness: Building Resilience in a Challenging Institutional Context," *American Psychologist*, Vol. 66, No. 1, 2011, pp. 4–9. As of September 26, 2014:
http://www.ncbi.nlm.nih.gov/pubmed/21219042

Costigan, S. A., L. Barnett, R. C. Plotnikoff, and D. R. Lubans, "The Health Indicators Associated with Screen-Based Sedentary Behavior Among Adolescent Girls: A Systematic

Review," *Journal of Adolescent Health*, Vol. 52, No. 4, April 2013, pp. 382–2013. As of September 26, 2014:
http://www.ncbi.nlm.nih.gov/pubmed/23299000

Damiani, G., L. Pinnarelli, S. C. Colosimo, R. Almiento, L. Sicuro, R. Galasso, L. Sommella, and W. Ricciardi, "The Effectiveness of Computerized Clinical Guidelines in the Process of Care: A Systematic Review," *BMC Health Services Research*, Vol. 10, 2010, p. 2. As of September 26, 2014:
http://www.ncbi.nlm.nih.gov/pubmed/20047686

Dayer, L., S. Heldenbrand, P. Anderson, P. O. Gubbins, and B. C. Martin, "Smartphone Medication Adherence Apps: Potential Benefits to Patients and Providers," *Journal of the American Pharmacists Association*, Vol. 53, No. 2, March–April 2013, pp. 172–181.

Devries, K. M., J. Y. Mak, L. J. Bacchus, J. C. Child, G. Falder, M. Petzold, J. Astbury, and C. H. Watts, "Intimate Partner Violence and Incident Depressive Symptoms and Suicide Attempts: A Systematic Review of Longitudinal Studies," *PLoS Medicine*, Vol. 10, No. 5, 2013. As of September 26, 2014:
http://www.ncbi.nlm.nih.gov/pubmed/23671407

Dietrich, Sandra, Stefanie Deckert, Martin Ceynowa, Ulrich Hegerl, and Katarina Stengler, "Depression in the Workplace: A Systematic Review of Evidence-Based Prevention Strategies," *International Archives of Occupational and Environmental Health*, Vol. 85, No. 1, 2012, pp. 1–11.

DoD—*see* U.S. Department of Defense.

Donker, T., K. Petrie, J. Proudfoot, J. Clarke, M. R. Birch, and H. Christensen, "Smartphones for Smarter Delivery of Mental Health Programs: A Systematic Review," *Journal of Medical Internet Research*, Vol. 15, No. 11, November 2013.

Dowling, Mitchell, and Debra Rickwood, "Online Counseling and Therapy for Mental Health Problems: A Systematic Review of Individual Synchronous Interventions Using Chat," *Journal of Technology in Human Services*, Vol. 31, No. 1, 2013, pp. 1–21.

Eidelson, R., M. Pilisuk, and S. Soldz, "The Dark Side of Comprehensive Soldier Fitness," *American Psychologist*, Vol. 66, No. 7, October 2011, pp. 643–644, 646–647. As of September 26, 2014:
http://www.ncbi.nlm.nih.gov/pubmed/21967209

Eysenbach, G., "The Law of Attrition," *Journal of Medical Internet Research*, Vol. 7, No. 1, January–March 2005.

Fann, J. R., D. L. Berry, S. Wolpin, M. Austin-Seymour, N. Bush, B. Halpenny, W. B. Lober, and R. McCorkle, "Depression Screening Using the Patient Health Questionnaire-9

Administered on a Touch Screen Computer," *Psychooncology*, Vol. 18, No. 1, 2009, pp. 14–22.

Fiordelli, M., N. Diviani, and P. J. Schulz, "Mapping mHealth Research: A Decade of Evolution," *Journal of Medical Internet Research*, Vol. 15, No. 4, 2013, p. e95.

Foran, H. M., and K. D. O'Leary, "Alcohol and Intimate Partner Violence: A Meta-Analytic Review," *Clinical Psychology Review*, Vol. 28, No. 7, October 2008, pp. 1222–1234. As of September 26, 2014: http://www.ncbi.nlm.nih.gov/pubmed/18550239

Fortney, J. C., J. M. Pyne, M. J. Edlund, D. K. Williams, D. E. Robinson, D. Mittal, and K. L. Henderson, "A Randomized Trial of Telemedicine-Based Collaborative Care for Depression," *Journal of General Internal Medicine*, Vol. 22, No. 8, August 2007, pp. 1086–1093.

Fortney, J. C., J. M. Pyne, S. B. Mouden, D. Mittal, T. J. Hudson, G. W. Schroeder, D. K. Williams, C. A. Bynum, R. Mattox, and K. M. Rost, "Practice-Based Versus Telemedicine-Based Collaborative Care for Depression in Rural Federally Qualified Health Centers: A Pragmatic Randomized Comparative Effectiveness Trial," *American Journal of Psychiatry*, Vol. 170, No. 4, April 2013, pp. 414–425.

Fowler, D. N., and M. Faulkner, "Interventions Targeting Substance Abuse Among Women Survivors of Intimate Partner Abuse: A Meta-Analysis," *Journal of Substance Abuse Treatment*, Vol. 41, No. 4, December 2011, pp. 386–398. As of September 26, 2014: http://www.ncbi.nlm.nih.gov/pubmed/21757316

Foxcroft, D. R., and A. Tsertsvadze, "Universal Multi-Component Prevention Programs for Alcohol Misuse in Young People," *Cochrane Database of Systematic Reviews*, No. 9, September 2011. As of September 30, 2014: http://www.ncbi.nlm.nih.gov/pubmed/21901732

Free, C., G. Phillips, L. Galli, L. Watson, L. Felix, P. Edwards, V. Patel, and A. Haines, "The Effectiveness of Mobile-Health Technology-Based Health Behaviour Change or Disease Management Interventions for Health Care Consumers: A Systematic Review," *PLoS Medicine*, Vol. 10, No. 1, 2013, p. e1001362. As of September 26, 2014: http://www.ncbi.nlm.nih.gov/pubmed/23349621

Frieden, T. R., "A Framework for Public Health Action: The Health Impact Pyramid," *American Journal of Public Health*, Vol. 100, No. 4, 2010, pp. 590–595.

Frueh, B. C., S. Henderson, and H. Myrick, "Telehealth Service Delivery for Persons with Alcoholism," *Journal of Telemedicine and Telecare*, Vol. 11, No. 7, 2005, pp. 372–375.

Frueh, B. C., J. Monnier, E. Yim, A. L. Grubaugh, M. B. Hamner, and R. G. Knapp, "A Randomized Trial of Telepsychiatry for Post-Traumatic Stress Disorder," *Journal of Telemedicine and Telecare*, Vol. 13, No. 3, 2007, pp. 142–147.

Garg, A. X., N. K. Adhikari, H. McDonald, M. P. Rosas-Arellano, P. J. Devereaux, J. Beyene, J. Sam, and R. B. Haynes, "Effects of Computerized Clinical Decision Support Systems on Practitioner Performance and Patient Outcomes: A Systematic Review," *JAMA: The Journal of the American Medical Association*, Vol. 293, No. 10, March 9, 2005, pp. 1223–1238. As of September 26, 2014: http://www.ncbi.nlm.nih.gov/pubmed/15755945

Germain, V., A. Marchand, S. Bouchard, M. S. Drouin, and S. Guay, "Effectiveness of Cognitive Behavioural Therapy Administered by Videoconference for Posttraumatic Stress Disorder," *Cognitive Behavioral Therapy*, Vol. 38, No. 1, 2009, pp. 42–53. As of September 26, 2014: http://www.ncbi.nlm.nih.gov/pubmed/19235601

Gilbody, S., P. Whitty, J. Grimshaw, and R. Thomas, "Educational and Organizational Interventions to Improve the Management of Depression in Primary Care: A Systematic Review," *JAMA: The Journal of the American Medical Association*, Vol. 289, No. 23, 2003, pp. 3145–3151.

Godard, C., A. Chevalier, Y. Lecrubier, and G. Lahon, "APRAND Programme: An Intervention to Prevent Relapses of Anxiety and Depressive Disorders: First Results of a Medical Health Promotion Intervention in a Population of Employees," *European Psychiatry*, Vol. 21, No. 7, 2006, pp. 451–459.

Golkaramnay, V., S. Bauer, S. Haug, M. Wolf, and H. Kordy, "The Exploration of the Effectiveness of Group Therapy Through an Internet Chat as Aftercare: A Controlled Naturalistic Study," *Psychotherapy and Psychosomatics*, Vol. 76, No. 4, 2007, pp. 219–225. As of September 26, 2014: http://www.ncbi.nlm.nih.gov/pubmed/17570960

Haynes, R. B., H. P. McDonald, and A. X. Garg, "Helping Patients Follow Prescribed Treatment: Clinical Applications," *JAMA: The Journal of the American Medical Association*, Vol. 288, No. 22, December 11, 2002, pp. 2880–2883. As of September 26, 2014: http://www.ncbi.nlm.nih.gov/pubmed/12472330

Hedman, E., G. Andersson, B. Ljotsson, E. Andersson, C. Ruck, E. Mortberg, and N. Lindefors, "Internet-Based Cognitive Behavior Therapy vs. Cognitive Behavioral Group Therapy for Social Anxiety Disorder: A Randomized Controlled Non-Inferiority Trial," *PLoS One*, Vol. 6, No. 3, 2011, p. e18001. As of September 26, 2014: http://www.ncbi.nlm.nih.gov/pubmed/21483704

Hertlein, Katherine M., Markie L. C. Blumer, and Justin M. Smith, "Marriage and Family Therapists' Use and Comfort with Online Communication with Clients," *Contemporary Family Therapy*, Vol. 36, No. 1, 2014, pp. 58–69.

Hilty, D. M., D. C. Ferrer, M. B. Parish, B. Johnston, E. J. Callahan, and P. M. Yellowlees, "The Effectiveness of Telemental Health: A 2013 Review," *Telemedicine and E-Health*, Vol. 19, No. 6, June 2013, pp. 444–454.

Hofmann, S. G., A. Asnaani, I. J. Vonk, A. T. Sawyer, and A. Fang, "The Efficacy of Cognitive Behavioral Therapy: A Review of Meta-Analyses," *Cognitive Therapy and Research*, Vol. 36, No. 5, October 1, 2012, pp. 427–440. As of September 26, 2014: http://www.ncbi.nlm.nih.gov/pubmed/23459093

Hunsley, John, Katherine Elliott, and Zoé Therrien, "The Efficacy and Effectiveness of Psychological Treatments for Mood, Anxiety, and Related Disorders," *Canadian Psychology/Psychologie Canadienne*, Vol. 55, No. 3, 2014, pp. 161–176.

Institute of Medicine, *Preventing Psychological Disorders in Service Members and Their Families: An Assessment of Programs*, Washington, D.C.: National Academies Press, February 2014. As of September 26, 2014: http://www.ncbi.nlm.nih.gov/books/NBK222170/

IoM—*see* Institute of Medicine.

Jaspers, M. W., M. Smeulers, H. Vermeulen, and L. W. Peute, "Effects of Clinical Decision-Support Systems on Practitioner Performance and Patient Outcomes: A Synthesis of High-Quality Systematic Review Findings," *Journal of the American Medical Informatics Association*, Vol. 18, No. 3, May 1, 2011, pp. 327–334. As of September 26, 2014: http://www.ncbi.nlm.nih.gov/pubmed/21422100

Jonsson U., I. Alaie, T. Parling, and F. K. Arnberg, "Reporting of Harms in Randomized Controlled Trials of Psychological Interventions for Mental and Behavioral Disorders: A Review of Current Practice," *Contemporary Clinical Trials*, Vol. 38, No. 1, May 2014, pp. 1–8. As of September 26, 2014: http://www.ncbi.nlm.nih.gov/pubmed/24607768

Kelders, S. M., R. N. Kok, H. C. Ossebaard, and J. E. Van Gemert-Pijnen, "Persuasive System Design Does Matter: A Systematic Review of Adherence to Web-Based Interventions," *Journal of Medical Internet Research*, Vol. 14, No. 6, 2012, p. e152. As of September 26, 2014: http://www.ncbi.nlm.nih.gov/pubmed/23151820

Kim, E. H., A. Coumar, W. B. Lober, and Y. Kim, "Addressing Mental Health Epidemic Among University Students via Web-Based, Self-Screening, and Referral System: A Preliminary

Study," *IEEE Transactions on Information Technology in Biomedicine: A Publication of the IEEE Engineering in Medicine and Biology Society*, Vol. 15. No. 2, 2011, pp. 301–307.

Klasnja, P., and W. Pratt, "Healthcare in the Pocket: Mapping the Space of Mobile-Phone Health Interventions," *Journal of Biomedical Informatics*, Vol. 45, No. 1, 2012, pp. 184–198.Kobak, K. A., L. H. Taylor, S. L. Dottl, J. H. Greist, J. W. Jefferson, D. Burroughs, D. J. Katzelnick, and M. Mandell, "Computerized Screening for Psychiatric Disorders in an Outpatient Community Mental Health Clinic," *Psychiatric Services*, Vol. 48, No. 8, August 1997, pp. 1048–1057.

Kravitz, R. L., P. Franks, M. D. Feldman, D. J. Tancredi, C. A. Slee, R. M. Epstein, P. R. Duberstein, R. A. Bell, M. Jackson-Triche, D. A. Paterniti, C. Cipri, A. M. Iosif, S. Olson, S. Kelly-Reif, A. Hudnut, S. Dvorak, C. Turner, and A. Jerant, "Patient Engagement Programs for Recognition and Initial Treatment of Depression in Primary Care: A Randomized Trial," *JAMA: The Journal of the Americal Medical Association*, Vol. 310, No. 17, November 6, 2013, pp. 1818–1828. As of September 26, 2014: http://www.ncbi.nlm.nih.gov/pubmed/24193079

Krishna, S., S. A. Boren, and E. A. Balas, "Healthcare via Cell Phones: A Systematic Review," *Telemedicine and E-Health: The Official Journal of the American Telemedicine Association*, Vol. 15, No. 3, 2009, pp. 231–240.

Kuhn, E., A. Eftekhari, J. E. Hoffman, J. J. Crowley, K. M. Ramsey, G. M. Reger, and J. I. Ruzek, "Clinician Perceptions of Using a Smartphone App with Prolonged Exposure Therapy," *Adminstration and Policy in Mental Health*, epub January 8, 2014. As of September 26, 2014:
http://www.ncbi.nlm.nih.gov/pubmed/24398700

Lapham, G. T., C. E. Achtmeyer, E. C. Williams, E. J. Hawkins, D. R. Kivlahan, and K. A. Bradley, "Increased Documented Brief Alcohol Interventions with a Performance Measure and Electronic Decision Support," *Medical Care*, Vol. 50, No. 2, February 2012, pp. 179–187. As of September 26, 2014:
http://www.ncbi.nlm.nih.gov/pubmed/20881876

Lawley, Jeffrey S., "HIPAA, HITECH and the Practicing Counselor: Electronic Records and Practice Guidelines," *The Professional Counselor*, Vol. 2, No. 3, 2012, pp. 192–200.

Lawrence, S. T., J. H. Willig, H. M. Crane, J. Ye, I. Aban, W. Lober, C. R. Nevin, D. S. Batey, M. J. Mugavero, C. McCullumsmith, C. Wright, M. Kitahata, J. L. Raper, M. S. Saag, and J. E. Schumacher, "Routine, Self-Administered, Touch-Screen, Computer-Based Suicidal Ideation Assessment Linked to Automated Response Team Notification in an HIV Primary Care Setting," *Clinical Infectious Diseases*, Vol. 50, No. 8, 2010, pp. 1165–1173.

Lester, P. B., P. D. Harms, M. N. Herian, D. V. Krasikova, and S. J. Beal, *The Comprehensive Soldier Fitness Program Evaluation, Report #3: Longitudinal Analysis of the Impact of Master Resilience Training on Self-Reported Resilience and Psychological Health Data*, Washington, D.C.: Department of Defense, 2011. As of September 12, 2014: http://www.dtic.mil/cgi-bin/GetTRDoc?Location=U2&doc=GetTRDoc.pdf&AD=ADA553635

Luxton, D. D., R. A. McCann, N. E. Bush, M. C. Mishkind, and G. M. Reger, "mHealth for Mental Health: Integrating Smartphone Technology in Behavioral Healthcare," *Professional Psychology: Research and Practice*, Vol. 42, No. 6, 2011, p. 505.

Mayou, R. A., A. Ehlers, and M. Hobbs, "Psychological Debriefing for Road Traffic Accident Victims. Three-Year Follow-Up of a Randomised Controlled Trial," *The British Journal of Psychiatry*, Vol. 176, June 2000, pp. 589–593. As of September 26, 2014: http://www.ncbi.nlm.nih.gov/pubmed/10974967

McKay, J. R., D. H. Van Horn, D. W. Oslin, K. G. Lynch, M. Ivey, K. Ward, M. L. Drapkin, J. R. Becher, and D. M. Coviello, "A Randomized Trial of Extended Telephone-Based Continuing Care for Alcohol Dependence: Within-Treatment Substance Use Outcomes," *Journal of Consulting and Clinical Psychology*, Vol. 78, No. 6, December 2010, pp. 912–923. As of September 26, 2014: http://www.ncbi.nlm.nih.gov/pubmed/20873894

McKeanna, M. T., C. M. Michaud, C. J. Murray, and J. S. Marks, "Assessing the Burden of Disease in the United States Using Disability-Adjusted Life Years," *American Journal of Preventive Medicine*, Vol. 28, No. 5, June 2005, pp. 415–423. As of September 26, 2014: http://www.ncbi.nlm.nih.gov/pubmed/15894144

Messer, S. C., X. Liu, C. W. Hoge, D. N. Cowan, and C. C. Engel, Jr., "Projecting Mental Disorder Prevalence from National Surveys to Populations-of-Interest—An Illustration Using ECA Data and the U. S. Army," *Social Psychiatry Psychiatric Epidemiology*, Vol. 39, No. 6, June 2004, pp. 419–426. As of September 26, 2014: http://www.ncbi.nlm.nih.gov/pubmed/15205725

Miller, C. W., and S. Himelhoch, "Acceptability of Mobile Phone Technology for Medication Adherence Interventions Among HIV-Positive Patients at an Urban Clinic," *AIDS Research and Treatment*, epub August 13, 2013, p. 670525. As of September 26, 2014: http://www.ncbi.nlm.nih.gov/pubmed/23997948

Miller, Laura L., Laurie T. Martin, Douglas Yeung, Matthew Trujillo, and Martha J. Timmer, *Information and Communication Technologies to Promote Social and Psychological Well-Being in the Air Force: A 2012 Survey of Airmen*, Santa Monica, Calif.: RAND Corporation,

RR-695-AF, 2014. As of April 2, 2015:
http://www.rand.org/pubs/research_reports/RR695.html

Mohr, D. C., M. N. Burns, S. M. Schueller, G. Clarke, and M. Klinkman, "Behavioral Intervention Technologies: Evidence Review and Recommendations for Future Research in Mental Health," *General Hospital Psychiatry*, Vol. 35, No. 4, 2013a, pp. 332–338.

Mohr, David C, Ken Cheung, Stephen M. Schueller, C. Hendricks Brown, and Naihua Duan, "Continuous Evaluation of Evolving Behavioral Intervention Technologies," *American Journal of Preventive Medicine*, Vol. 45, No. 4, 2013b, pp. 517–523.

Moreira, M. T., L. A. Smith, and D. Foxcroft, "Social Norms Interventions to Reduce Alcohol Misuse in University or College Students," *Cochrane Database of Systematic Reviews*, Vol. 3, July 2009. As of September 26, 2014:
http://www.ncbi.nlm.nih.gov/pubmed/19588402

Moreno, F. A., J. Chong, J. Dumbauld, M. Humke, and S. Byreddy, "Use of Standard Webcam and Internet Equipment for Telepsychiatry Treatment of Depression Among Underserved Hispanics," *Psychiatric Services*, Vol. 63, No. 12, December 2012, pp. 1213–1217.

Morland, L. A., C. J. Greene, C. S. Rosen, D. Foy, P. Reilly, J. Shore, Q. M. He, and B. C. Frueh, "Telemedicine for Anger Management Therapy in a Rural Population of Combat Veterans With Posttraumatic Stress Disorder: A Randomized Noninferiority Trial,"*Journal of Clinical Psychiatry*, Vol. 71, No. 7, July 2010, pp. 855–863.

Muñoz, Ricardo F., Pim Cuijpers, Filip Smit, Alinne Z. Barrera, and Yan Leykin, "Prevention of Major Depression," *Annual Review of Clinical Psychology*, Vol. 6, 2010, pp. 181–212. As of September 26, 2014:
http://www.ncbi.nlm.nih.gov/pubmed/20192789

Murdoch, J. W., and P. A. Connor-Greene, "Enhancing Therapeutic Impact and Therapeutic Alliance Through Electronic Mail Homework Assignments," *Journal of Psychotherapy Practice and Research*, Vol. 9, No. 4, Fall 2000, pp. 232–237. As of September 26, 2014:
http://www.ncbi.nlm.nih.gov/pubmed/11069136

Musen, Mark A., Blackford Middleton, and Robert A. Greenes, "Clinical Decision-Support Systems," *Biomedical Informatics*, Spring 2014, pp. 643–674.

Myers, K., S. Cain, Work Group on Quality Issues, and American Academy of Child and Adolescent Psychiatry Staff, "Practice Parameter for Telepsychiatry with Children and Adolescents," *Journal of the American Academy of Child and Adolescent Psychiatry*, Vol. 47, No. 12, December 2008, pp. 1468–1483. As of September 26, 2014:
http://www.ncbi.nlm.nih.gov/pubmed/19034191

Newman, M. G., L. E. Szkodny, S. J. Llera, and A. Przeworski, "A Review of Technology-Assisted Self-Help and Minimal Contact Therapies for Anxiety and Depression: Is Human Contact Necessary for Therapeutic Efficacy?" *Clinical Psychology Review*, Vol. 31, No. 1, February 2011, pp. 89–103. As of September 26, 2014: http://www.ncbi.nlm.nih.gov/pubmed/21130939

Newton, N. C., G. Andrews, K. E. Champion, and M. Teesson, "Universal Internet-Based Prevention for Alcohol and Cannabis Use Reduces Truancy, Psychological Distress and Moral Disengagement: A Cluster Randomised Controlled Trial," *Preventive Medicine*, Vol. 65, August 2014a, pp. 109–115. As of September 26, 2014: http://www.ncbi.nlm.nih.gov/pubmed/24823906

Newton, N. C., P. J. Conrod, D. M. Rodriguez, and M. Teesson, "A Pilot Study of an Online Universal School-Based Intervention to Prevent Alcohol and Cannabis Use in the UK," *BMJ Open*, May 2014b. As of September 26, 2014: http://www.ncbi.nlm.nih.gov/pubmed/24840248

Newton, N. C., M. Teesson, L. E. Vogl, and G. Andrews, "Internet-Based Prevention for Alcohol and Cannabis Use: Final Results of the Climate Schools Course," *Addiction*, Vol. 105, No. 4, April 2010, pp. 749–759. As of September 20, 2014: http://www.ncbi.nlm.nih.gov/pubmed/20148791

Pelosi, A. J., and G. Lewis, "The Computer Will See You Now," *BMJ,* Vol. 299, No. 6692, July 15, 1989, pp. 138–139. As of September 26, 2014: http://www.ncbi.nlm.nih.gov/pubmed/2504350

Pew Research Internet Project, "Mobile Technology Fact Sheet," 2014. As of September 25, 2014: http://www.pewinternet.org/fact-sheets/mobile-technology-fact-sheet/

Powell, B. J., J. C. McMillen, E. K. Proctor, C. R. Carpenter, R. T. Griffey, A. C. Bunger, J. E. Glass, and J. L. York, "A Compilation of Strategies for Implementing Clinical Innovations in Health and Mental Health," *Medical Care Research and Review*, Vol. 69, No. 2, April 2012, pp. 123–157. As of September 26, 2014: http://www.ncbi.nlm.nih.gov/pubmed/22203646

Price, Matthew, Kenneth J. Ruggiero, Pamela L. Ferguson, Sachin K. Patel, Frank Treiber, Deborah Couillard, and Samir M. Fahkry, "A Feasibility Pilot Study on the Use of Text Messages to Track PTSD Symptoms After a Traumatic Injury," *General Hospital Psychiatry*, Vol. 36, No. 3, 2014, pp. 249–254. As of June 2014: http://www.sciencedirect.com/science/article/pii/S0163834314000541

Price, M., E. K. Yuen, E. M. Goetter, J. D. Herbert, E. M. Forman, R. Acierno, and K. J. Ruggiero, "mHealth: A Mechanism to Deliver More Accessible, More Effective Mental

Health Care," *Clinical Psychology & Psychotherapy*, August 5, 2013. As of September 26, 2014:
http://www.ncbi.nlm.nih.gov/pubmed/23918764

Richards, D., and T. Richardson, "Computer-Based Psychological Treatments for Depression: A Systematic Review and Meta-Analysis," *Clinical Psychology Review*, Vol. 32, No. 4, June 2012, pp. 329–342. As of September 26, 2014:
http://www.ncbi.nlm.nih.gov/pubmed/22466510

Riper H., A. van Straten, M. Keuken, F. Smit, G. Schippers, and P. Cuijpers, "Curbing Problem Drinking with Personalized-Feedback Interventions: A Meta-Analysis," *American Journal of Preventitive Medicine*, Vol. 36, No. 3, March 2009, pp. 247–255. As of September 26, 2014:
http://www.ncbi.nlm.nih.gov/pubmed/19215850

Ritterband, L. M., F. P. Thorndike, L. A. Gonder-Frederick, J. C. Magee, E. T. Bailey, D. K. Saylor, and C. M. Morin, "Efficacy of an Internet-Based Behavioral Intervention for Adults with Insomnia," *Archives of General Psychiatry*, Vol. 66, No. 7, July 2009, pp. 692–698. As of September 26, 2014:
http://www.ncbi.nlm.nih.gov/pubmed/19581560

Roberts, N. P., N. J. Kitchiner, J. Kenardy, and J. Bisson, "Multiple Session Early Psychological Interventions for the Prevention of Post-Traumatic Stress Disorder," *Cochrane Database of Systematic Review*, Vol. 3, July 8, 2009. As of September 26, 2014:
http://www.ncbi.nlm.nih.gov/pubmed/19588408

Robertson, L., M. Smith, D. Castle, and D. Tannenbaum, "Using the Internet to Enhance the Treatment of Depression," *Australas Psychiatry*, Vol. 14, No. 4, December 2006, pp. 413–417. As of September 26, 2014:
http://www.ncbi.nlm.nih.gov/pubmed/17116083

Robinson, S., S. Perkins, S. Bauer, N. Hammond, J. Treasure, and U. Schmidt, "Aftercare Intervention Through Text Messaging in the Treatment of Bulimia Nervosa—Feasibility Pilot," *International Journal of Eating Disorders*, Vol. 39, No. 8, December 2006, pp. 633–638. As of September 26, 2014:
http://www.ncbi.nlm.nih.gov/pubmed/16937381

Rollman, B. L., B. H. Hanusa, H. J. Lowe, T. Gilbert, W. N. Kapoor, and H. C. Schulberg, "A Randomized Trial Using Computerized Decision Support to Improve Treatment of Major Depression in Primary Care," *Journal of General Internal Medicine*, Vol. 17, No. 7, July 2002, pp. 493–503. As of September 26, 2014:
http://www.ncbi.nlm.nih.gov/pubmed/12133139

Romano, M. J., and R. S. Stafford, "Electronic Health Records and Clinical Decision Support Systems: Impact on National Ambulatory Care Quality," *Archives of Internal Medicine*, Vol.

171, No. 10, May 23, 2011, pp. 897–903. As of September 26, 2014: http://www.ncbi.nlm.nih.gov/pubmed/21263077

Rona, R. J., K. C. Hyams, and S. Wessely, "Screening for Psychological Illness in Military Personnel," *JAMA: The Journal of the American Medical Association*, Vol. 293, No. 10, March 2005, pp. 1257–1260.

Rooke, S., E. Thorsteinsson, A. Karpin, J. Copeland, and D. Allsop, "Computer-Delivered Interventions for Alcohol and Tobacco Use: A Meta-Analysis," *Addiction*, Vol. 105, No. 8, August 2010, pp. 1381–1390. As of September 26, 2014: http://www.ncbi.nlm.nih.gov/pubmed/20528806

Ruskin, P. E., M. Silver-Aylaian, M. A. Kling, S. A. Reed, D. D. Bradham, J. R. Hebel, D. Barrett, F. Knowles, and P. Hauser, "Treatment Outcomes in Depression: Comparison of Remote Treatment Through Telepsychiatry to In-Person Treatment," *American Journal of Psychiatry*, Vol. 161, No. 8, August 2004, pp. 1471–1476.

Santiago, P. N., J. E. Wilk, C. S. Milliken, C. A. Castro, C. C. Engel, and C. W. Hoge, "Screening for Alcohol Misuse and Alcohol-Related Behaviors Among Combat Veterans," *Psychiatric Services*, Vol. 61, No. 6, June 2010, pp. 575–581. As of September 26, 2014: http://www.ncbi.nlm.nih.gov/pubmed/20513680

Sleep Healthy Using the Internet, home page, 2013. As of September 26, 2014: http://www.shuti.net

Smith, G. S., C. C. Branas, and T. R. Miller, "Fatal Nontraffic Injuries Involving Alcohol: A Metaanalysis," *Annals of Emergency Medicine*, Vol. 33, No. 6, June 1999, pp. 659–668. As of September 26, 2014: http://www.ncbi.nlm.nih.gov/pubmed/10339681

Smith, S. L., "Could Comprehensive Soldier Fitness Have Iatrogenic Consequences? A Commentary," *Journal of Behavioral Health Services and Research*, Vol. 40, No. 2, April 2013, pp. 242–246. As of September 26, 2014: http://www.ncbi.nlm.nih.gov/pubmed/23229522

Steenkamp, M. M., W. P. Nash, and B. T. Litz, "Post-Traumatic Stress Disorder: Review of the Comprehensive Soldier Fitness Program," *American Journal of Preventive Medicine*, Vol. 44, No. 5, 2013, pp. 507–512. As of September 26, 2014: http://www.ncbi.nlm.nih.gov/pubmed/23597815

Swigert, T. J., M. W. True, T. J. Sauerwein, and H. Dai, "U.S. Air Force Telehealth Initiative to Assist Primary Care Providers in the Management of Diabetes," *Clinical Diabetes*, Vol. 32, No. 2, 2014, pp. 78–80.

Teesson, M., N. C. Newton, T. Slade, C. Chapman, S. Allsop, L. Hides, N. McBride, L. M. Newton, A. Tonks, L. Birrell, L. Brownhill, and G. Andrews, "The CLIMATE Schools

Combined Study: A Cluster Randomised Controlled Trial of a Universal Internet-Based Prevention Program for Youth Substance Misuse, Depression and Anxiety," *BMC Psychiatry*, Vol. 14, No. 32, February 5, 2014. As of September 29, 2014: http://www.ncbi.nlm.nih.gov/pubmed/24499060

Thorndike, F.P., L. M. Ritterband, L. A. Gonder-Frederick, H, R. Lord, K. S. Ingersoll, and C. M. Morin, "A Randomized Controlled Trial of an Internet Intervention for Adults with Insomnia: Effects on Comorbid Psychological and Fatigue Symptoms," *Journal of Clinical Psychology*, Vol. 69, No. 10, October 2013, pp. 1078–1093. As of September 26, 2014: http://www.ncbi.nlm.nih.gov/pubmed/24014057

Tomlinson, M., M. J. Rotheram-Borus, L. Swartz, and A. C. Tsai, "Scaling Up mHealth: Where Is the Evidence?" *PLoS Medicine*, Vol. 10, No. 2, 2013, p. e1001382. As of September 26, 2014: http://www.ncbi.nlm.nih.gov/pubmed/23424286

Turvey, C., M. Coleman, O. Dennison, K. Drude, M. Goldenson, P. Hirsch, R. Jueneman, G. M. Kramer, D. D. Luxton, M. M. Maheu, T. S. Malik, M. C. Mishkind, T. Rabinowitz, L. J. Roberts, T. Sheeran, J. H. Shore, P. Shore, F. van Heeswyk, B. Wregglesworth, P. Yellowlees, M. L. Zucker, E. A. Krupinski, and J. Bernard, "ATA Practice Guidelines for Video-Based Online Mental Health Services," *Telemedicine and E-Health*, Vol. 19, No. 9, September 2013, pp. 722–730. As of September 26, 2014: http://www.ncbi.nlm.nih.gov/pubmed/23909884

Unützer, J., Y. Choi, I. A. Cook, and S. Oishi, "A Web-Based Data Management System to Improve Care for Depression in a Multicenter Clinical Trial," *Psychiatric Services*, Vol. 53, No. 6, June 2002a, pp. 671–673, 678. As of September 26, 2014: http://www.ncbi.nlm.nih.gov/pubmed/12045303

Unützer, J., W. Katon, C. M. Callahan, J. W. Williams, Jr., E. Hunkeler, L. Harpole, M. Hoffing, R. D. Della Penna, P. H. Noel, E. H. Lin, P. A. Arean, M. T. Hegel, L. Tang, T. R. Belin, S. Oishi, C. Langston, and IMPACT Investigators (Improving Mood-Promoting Access to Collaborative Treatment), "Collaborative Care Management of Late-Life Depression in the Primary Care Setting: A Randomized Controlled Trial," *JAMA: The Journal of the American Medical Association*, Vol. 288, No. 22, December 2002b, pp. 2836–2845. As of September 26, 2014: http://www.ncbi.nlm.nih.gov/pubmed/12472325

U.S. Department of Defense, *2012 Demographics: Profile of the Military Community*, Washington, D.C.: Office of the Deputy Assistant Secretary of Defense (Military Community and Family Policy), 2013. As of September 21, 2014: http://www.militaryonesource.mil/12038/MOS/Reports/2012-Demographics-Report.pdf

van Ballegooijen, W., P. Cuijpers, A. van Straten, E. Karyotaki, G. Andersson, J. H. Smit, and H. Riper, "Adherence to Internet-Based and Face-to-Face Cognitive Behavioural Therapy for Depression: A Meta-Analysis," *PLoS One*, Vol. 9, No. 7, 2014, p. e100674. As of September 26, 2014:
http://www.ncbi.nlm.nih.gov/pubmed/25029507

Varshney, U., "A Model for Improving Quality of Decisions in Mobile Health," *Decision Support Systems*, Vol. 62, June 2014, pp. 66–77.Varshney, U., "Mobile Health: Four Emerging Themes of Research," *Decision Support Systems*, Vol. 66, October 2014, pp. 20–35.

Wears, R. L., and M. Berg, "Computer Technology and Clinical Work: Still Waiting for Godot," *JAMA: The Journal of the American Medical Association*, Vol. 293, No. 10, March 9, 2005, pp. 1261–1263. As of September 26, 2014:
http://www.ncbi.nlm.nih.gov/pubmed/15755949

Weinick, R. M., E. B. Beckjord, C. M. Farmer, L. T. Martin, E. M. Gillen, J. D. Acosta, M. P. Fisher, J. Garnett, G. C. Gonzalez, T. C. Helmus, L. H. Jaycox, K. Reynolds, N. Salcedo, and D. M. Scharf, *Programs Addressing Psychological Health and Traumatic Brain Injury Among U.S. Military Servicemembers and Their Families*, Santa Monica, Calif.: RAND Corporation, TR-950-OSD, 2011. As of March 30, 2015:
http://www.rand.org/pubs/technical_reports/TR950.html

Welbourne, J. L., A. L. Blanchard, and M. B. Wadsworth, "Motivations in Virtual Health Communities and Their Relationship to Community, Connectedness and Stress," *Computers in Human Behavior*, Vol. 29, No. 1, 2013, pp.129–139.

Whiteford, H. A., L. Degenhardt, J. Rehm, A. J. Baxter, A. J. Ferrari, H. E. Erskine, F. J. Charlson, R. E. Norman, A. D. Flaxman, N. Johns, R. Burstein, C. J. Murray, and T. Vos, "Global Burden of Disease Attributable to Mental and Substance Use Disorders: Findings from the Global Burden of Disease Study 2010," *Lancet*, Vol. 382, No. 9904, November 2013, pp. 1575–1586. As of September 26, 2014:
http://www.ncbi.nlm.nih.gov/pubmed/23993280

Woltmann, E. M., S. M. Wilkniss, A. Teachout, G. J. McHugo, and R. E. Drake, "Trial of an Electronic Decision Support System to Facilitate Shared Decision Making in Community Mental Health," *Psychiatric Services*, Vol. 62, No. 1, January 2011, pp. 54–60. As of September 26, 2014:
http://www.ncbi.nlm.nih.gov/pubmed/21209300

Wood, S. K., L. Eckley, K. Hughes, K. A. Hardcastle, M. A. Bellis, J. Schrooten, Z. Demetrovics, and L. Voorham, "Computer-Based Programmes for the Prevention and Management of Illicit Recreational Drug Use: A Systematic Review," *Addictive Behaviors*, Vol. 39, No. 1, 2014, pp. 30–38.

Woodson, J., "Military Health System Introduces Telehealth Pilot Projects to Improve Access to Care," *U.S. Medicine*, July 2014. As of March 29, 2015: http://www.usmedicine.com/current-issue/military-health-system-introduces-telehealth-pilot-projects-to-improve-access-to-care/

Wright, A., J. Feblowitz, S. Phansalkar, J. Liu, A. Wilcox, C. A. Keohane, D. L. Seger, M. Bloomrosen, G. J. Kuperman, and D. W. Bates, "Preventability of Adverse Drug Events Involving Multiple Drugs Using Publicly Available Clinical Decision Support Tools," *American Journal of Health-System Pharmacy,* Vol. 69, No. 3, February 1, 2012, pp. 221–227. As of September 26, 2014: http://www.ncbi.nlm.nih.gov/pubmed/22261944

Yellowlees, P., J. Shore, L. Roberts, and American Telemedicine Association, "Practice Guidelines for Videoconferencing-Based Telemental Health—October 2009," *Telemedicine and E-Health*, Vol. 16, No. 10, December 2010, pp. 1074–1089. As of September 26, 2014: http://www.ncbi.nlm.nih.gov/pubmed/21186991